Disordered Minds

Williamsburg in America Series

VIII

The eighth in a series of popular histories
focusing on the roles of Williamsburg and Virginia
in the eighteenth century

Disordered Minds

The First Century of Eastern State Hospital in Williamsburg, Virginia 1766-1866

by

NORMAN DAIN

Published by
THE COLONIAL WILLIAMSBURG FOUNDATION
Williamsburg, Virginia

Distributed by
The University Press of Virginia
Charlottesville, Virginia

Library of Congress
Catalog Card Number: 76-135916

Colonial Williamsburg SBN: 910412-88-X
University Press of Virginia SBN: 8139-0317-3

Printed in the United States of America

FOR BRUCE

Table of Contents

List of Illustrations

Acknowledgments

IT is a pleasure to express thanks to those persons who have assisted my work on this book.

From Colonial Williamsburg I received financial support and complete cooperation. Working in Williamsburg was a delightful as well as fruitful experience. Dr. Edward P. Alexander, vice-president and director of the Division of Interpretation; Mr. James R. Short, assistant to Dr. Alexander; Mr. Joseph N. Rountree, director of publications; Mr. John J. Walklet, Jr., formerly director of publications; and Dr. Edward M. Riley, director of research, did all anyone could do to facilitate my work. To Mr. Short, Mr. Walklet, Mr. Rountree, Mr. Thomas K. Ford, editor of publications, and several anonymous readers I am indebted for valuable criticisms and suggestions and for meticulous editorial work. The entire staff of the Research Department offered warm hospitality and many kinds of assistance, most especially Dr. Riley, whose advice and wisdom were indispensable to me. Also at the Research Department I wish to thank particularly Mrs. Rose Belk, the librarian; Mrs. Marylee McGregor, the research archivist; and Miss Cornelia Fitzgerald, who handled my Xeroxing problems so efficiently. Dr. George H. Reese, then assistant director of research, was of aid in Dr. Riley's absence, and Mrs. Mary Goodwin was good enough to offer editorial comments and corrections. The extensive bibliographical and biographical study of the Eastern State Hospital that Mr. Junius Fishburne did under the supervision of the Research Department in preparation for my work was extremely helpful.

Through the courtesy of Dr. Howard H. Ashbury, superintendent of the Eastern State Hospital, and the assistance of the medical librarian, Mrs. Marjorie Caldwell, I was able to examine and have reproduced archival materials in the hospital. The former superintendent of the Western State Hospital at Staunton, Dr. James Druff, kindly allowed me to see archival materials there. At the College of William and Mary, Williamsburg, Mr. James Renz, then acting librarian, extended the courtesy of the library to me. Miss Margaret Cook, curator of manuscripts, was particularly helpful in locating manuscripts and rare books, and Mrs. Anna B. Johnson, the law librarian, gave me free access to the law collection and took care of reproducing various documents for me. The Virginia State Library's holdings of state documents and archives were invaluable to this study. Mr. M. C. Russell, head of the Reference and Circulation Section, and Mr. J. W. Dudley of the Archives greatly facilitated my search for materials. At the University of Virginia, Charlottesville, Mr. Edmund Berkeley of the Manuscript Division was most obliging, as was the staff of the Virginia Historical Society, Richmond. Mr. Elmer Parker of the Old Military Records Division of the National Archives unearthed records that illuminate the history of the Eastern State Hospital during the Civil War.

My research assistant at Rutgers University, Mr. Gary Stein, proofread part of the manuscript, and Mrs. Shirley Lerman and Mrs. Sarah Hope were the excellent typists.

Several friends read the book in manuscript and gave me useful suggestions: Dr. Eric T. Carlson of Cornell University Medical College–Payne Whitney Psychiatric Clinic; Dr. Gerald N. Grob of Rutgers University; and Dr. Barbara Sicherman of Manhattanville College. I would like also to thank the members of the Section on the History of Psychiatry and the Behavioral Sciences of the Department of Psychiatry, Cornell University Medical College, for their comments on talks that I gave describing this project.

I was enabled to finish the book through the generous award of a Research Council Faculty Fellowship from Rutgers University.

My wife, Dr. Phyllis Dain of Columbia University, is really a coauthor. She assisted me very materially in almost every stage of the manuscript's development. Her training in librarianship proved especially valuable in spying out new sources, and the entire manuscript benefited from her careful attention to organization and detail.

N. D.
Leonia, New Jersey
September, 1970

Introduction

MENTAL patients occupy about half the hospital beds in the United States. This often repeated figure (though it includes many persons not in need of psychiatric care and some not even mentally disordered) reflects success in compiling statistics and hospitalizing people but not in enabling them to live productive lives in the community at large. Our understanding of their troubles and knowledge of their proper treatment are still slight.

Attitudes in the western world toward mentally afflicted persons began only in the latter half of the eighteenth century to emerge from the obscurantism of the ages. To be sure, the past had not been one long benighted era unrelieved by rational psychiatric theories and compassionate care, but these were sporadic and selectively applied. In the eighteenth century, as never before, mental disorder, along with ills of all kinds, came under the scrutiny of influential thinkers and humanitarian activists—both medical and lay—as a medical and social problem to be dealt with by the total society. However, progress from cruelty or neglect to humane care, from ignorance to enlightenment, and from empiricism to science, has been far from steady. Advances, retrogressions, and renewed reform have characterized the past two centuries.

At the beginning of the new era of psychiatry the enlightened attitude toward mental patients was one of reform in their care and hope for their future. This spirit lasted, with some changes, for almost a century. It corresponded with a general burgeoning of optimism about man and his works that found expression in the American and French revolutions and in the successes in science and technology associated with the Industrial Revolution.

The people of British colonial America, or at least their political and intellectual leaders, partook of this spirit. Like their counterparts in England and Western Europe, some of them started programs to improve the condition of the disadvantaged and oppressed—the indigent sick, criminals, and insane; a few even talked about eliminating slavery and in time freed their own slaves. The largest colony and among the most influential, Virginia, with its widespread slave-worked plantations and small towns, did not produce many social thinkers and reformers but had its share of educated leaders with a sense of public responsibility. These men responded favorably to a call for a hospital to succor the mentally ill, the first one in the colonies devoted to this purpose alone and the first operated entirely under provincial or state auspices.

This hospital (hereafter called by its modern name, the Eastern State Hospital)* opened at Williamsburg, the capital of colonial Virginia, on October 12, 1773.† Twenty-two years before, the Pennsylvania Hospital in Philadelphia, the earliest functioning general hospital in what is now the United States, admitted insane patients.‡ But the Pennsylvania Hospital did not, so far as we know, inspire the founding of the Williamsburg institution. Local conditions and European influences rather than emulation of Philadelphia, then the leading colonial city, spurred Virginia to pioneer

---

* Before 1841 the Williamsburg asylum was called by many different names. The founding act of 1770 spoke of "a public hospital" and called the trustees the "court of directors of the public hospital, for persons of insane and disordered minds." In the act of March 6, 1841, the trustees were called "Directors of the Eastern Asylum for the maintenance and cure of insane persons." Then in March 1861 the legislature specifically named the hospital the Eastern Lunatic Asylum. Its current name, Eastern State Hospital, dates from 1894.

† The terms insane and insanity are today generally confined to courts of law, since the medical profession considers them inaccurate and misleading. During the eighteenth century and through most of the nineteenth, however, these terms were widely accepted within the profession as well as by the public. Other terms frequently used were lunatic, madman, and mentally deranged. None of these necessarily connoted hostility or ignorance on the part of those using them.

‡ Kentucky established at Lexington in 1824 the second state mental hospital (that is, if one excludes the complicated case of Spring Grove State Hospital, Catonsville, Maryland, opened in 1798). The second state hospital in Virginia, and the third in the United States, admitted patients in 1828. The first state hospital in the northern states, where corporate nonprofit institutions, sometimes with government support, were at first more common, was opened at Worcester, Massachusetts, in 1833.

in the treatment of the mentally ill. And local circumstances again helped to give the result of this effort, the Eastern State Hospital, some unique qualities, particularly through its first century, the best known being its management by one Williamsburg family, the Galts.

This study traces the hospital's history from its origin in the mid-1760s to the close of the Civil War. The disruptions of the war (in the South especially), changes in medicine and science, and various social and political conditions all combined to bring a renewed pessimism and neglect of the mentally ill in state hospitals, including the Eastern State Hospital. The Civil War years, then, marked not only that institution's approaching centennial but the abrupt end of the Galts' association with it and the breakdown of its therapeutic system. The story opens in the midst of a growing rebellion against colonial status; it closes at the end of a second and much more bitter fight over secession. Both struggles, one successful, the other ruinous, directly affected the hospital's fate, as they did, even more profoundly, the fate of society at large.

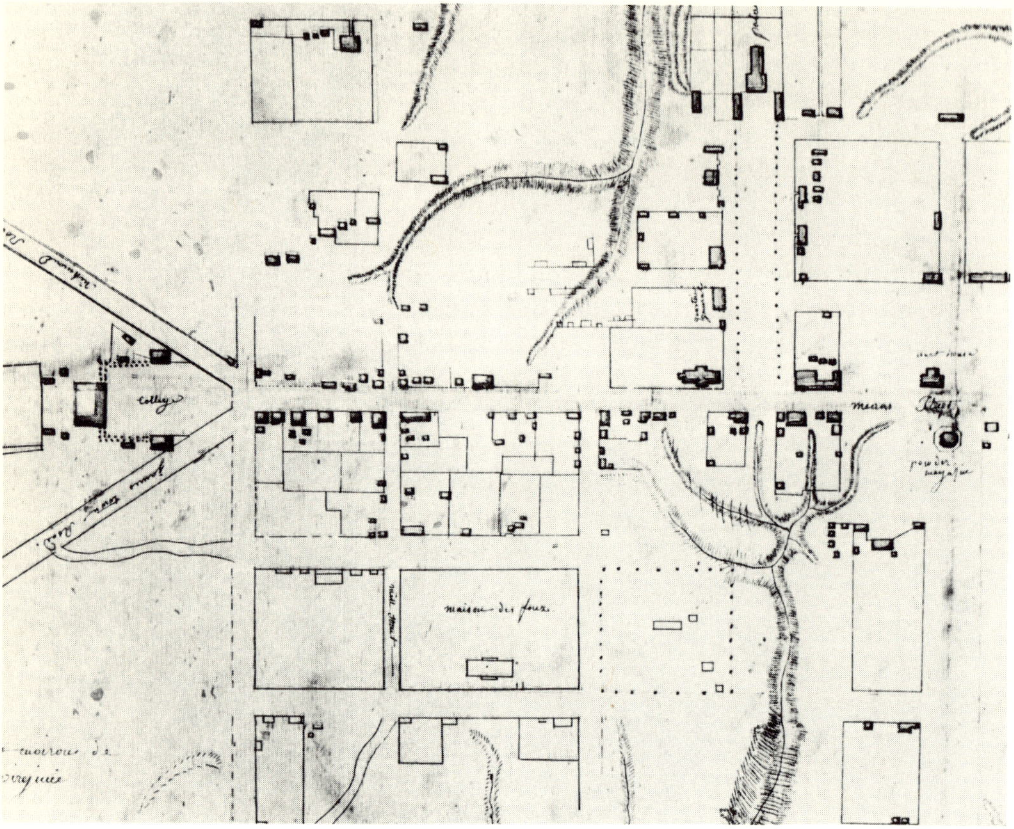

Figure 1
Map of Part of Williamsburg, 1782

A section from the "Frenchman's Map" of Williamsburg, showing the western part of the town and the relationship of the "Maison des foux" to the College of William and Mary (*left*) and the Courthouse and Powder Magazine (*right*).

CHAPTER ONE

The Founding and Early Years 1766-1800

[1]

EARLY in Virginia's history, colonial legislators concerned themselves with the legal status, rights, and property of the mentally incompetent and insane. Legislation passed in the 1660s concerning lawsuits, titles to lands, creditors' relief, unlawful hunting, and construction of water mills, for example, placed the insane under special protection, much like widows and orphans, as long as they remained non compos mentis. They were exempt from statutes of limitation or the execution of the law until they regained sane memory or sound mind.

As to the responsibility of insane defendants the situation was not so clear. In one case, occurring in 1661, legislators suspended, temporarily at least, the punishment of a man who slandered the king: "hee is disturbed in his braine, talking wildly and distractedly to such things as are put to him. . . ." During the same year the Virginia Assembly "*ordered* That Nicholas Perry be for the present released out of prison, and that he shall not be further prosecuted until wee have notice from the governour out of England next yeare whether a person in condition of a lunatick be suable or no." By the mid-eighteenth century the Virginia courts, like those in England, usually excluded some of the more obviously insane defendants from the penalties of the criminal law.

The last royal governor of Virginia, the earl of Dunmore, felt well satisfied with the legal provisions for the insane in his colony.

He could see no necessity for a new clause proposed in 1772 to be inserted by the Board of Trade "in the Commission for Governors of His Majesty's Colonies in America, giving them power to issue Commissions for the care and Custody of Ideots and Lunatics. . . ." He reported that "The method pursued in this Colony with respect to Ideots and Lunatics hath been conformable to the practise of the High Court of Chancery in England."

Cases would come before the colonial General Court, Dunmore explained, which would then issue a commission to the county sheriff commanding him to inquire of twelve citizens if the person involved was "a Lunatic or ideot." If he was found to be either, a proper person was appointed his committee or guardian, generally his next of kin but not his heir at law. Security was taken and an allowance settled on for his support and maintenance. The committee accounted to the court for the profits of the estate, as all guardians of orphans were obliged to do; the surplus, if any, was preserved for the "Lunatic" if he recovered a sound state of mind, or went after his death to those entitled to it. "There is perhaps no Country in the British Dominions, where persons under these unhappy circumstances are treated with more humanity, or are better taken care of." Dunmore was here referring to the mental hospital that had been authorized by law in 1770.

Until then the colony compared favorably with England in providing equity for the insane but had not shown particular concern for their safety, comfort, and treatment. As elsewhere in most of North America, the insane—if not cared for by family or friends, hired out to work for the lowest bidder, or supported by the church parish—languished in jails or were left to wander about the countryside.

The call for a mental hospital in Virginia had come from one of Dunmore's predecessors, Governor Francis Fauquier. An intellectually sophisticated, humane, and cultivated man, son of a French Huguenot who settled in England and prospered as a director of the Bank of England, Fauquier was considered one of Virginia's best royal governors. He was interested in science and, like his brother before him, had been honored by membership in the Royal Society. His concern for the plight of the insane seems to have originated in his enlightened views and a desire to protect the community.

Fauquier brought up the subject of a mental hospital on November 6, 1766, in his message to the opening session of the House of Burgesses, meeting for the first time since he had dissolved it nearly a year and a half before in response to the Stamp Act Resolves. After dwelling on the recent repeal of the Stamp Act as evidence of the affection the mother country had for her colonists, and appealing therefore for the latter's loyalty to the crown, Fauquier introduced an apparently unrelated issue:

> It is expedient I should also recommend to your Consideration and Humanity a poor unhappy set of People who are deprived of their Senses and wander about the Country, terrifying the Rest of their Fellow Creatures. A legal Confinement, and proper Provision, ought to be appointed for these miserable Objects, who cannot help themselves. Every civilized Country has an Hospital for these People, where they are confined, maintained and attended by able Physicians, to endeavour to restore to them their lost Reason.

That was all. Unlike the petitions Benjamin Franklin had drawn up in the campaign for the Pennsylvania Hospital, Fauquier discussed neither the dimensions of the problem of the insane in Virginia nor the advantages of hospital care as opposed to home care.

The burgesses responded favorably. On November 20 they passed a resolution calling for the erection of a mental hospital and designating the Committee of Propositions and Grievances to prepare the necessary bills. Then they dropped the matter. On April 11, 1767, at the end of the session, Fauquier spoke out again. The hospital bill, he said, "was a measure which I think could offend no party, and which I was in hopes humanity would have dictated to every man, as soon as he was made acquainted with the call for it." It was the burgesses' business, he reminded them, to provide for all sorts of poor people. Since he thought the hospital was of "some importance to the ease and comfort of the whole community, as well as a point of charity" to the insane, he intended to raise the issue again at the next session. His death the following March precluded that.

Fauquier's wish, however, was carried out. Eventually, on November 15, 1769, the burgesses ordered the Committee of Propositions and Grievances to draft appropriate legislation to provide for the mentally ill in the colony. Perhaps the interest of the new and equally popular and cultivated governor, Lord Botetourt, spurred them. Botetourt had already commissioned William Byrd III to ask the Pennsylvania Hospital to receive four insane persons imprisoned in Virginia.

The House of Burgesses officially heard on November 29 of the Pennsylvania Hospital's acquiescence, and the next day the members resolved "That an humble Address be presented to his Excellency the Governor, returning him the Thanks of this House" for his humane interest in the four unfortunates. His desire to send them temporarily to Philadelphia was approved, and the burgesses agreed to pay the necessary expenses until proper provision could be made for the insane in Virginia. Since the burgesses had moved favorably on the hospital two weeks before, the governor may have acted with full knowledge of their intensions, but it seems likely that he started negotiations with the Pennsylvania Hospital before the burgesses did anything specific.

The only obvious pressure other than from the two royal governors came from a single editorial in the *Virginia Gazette* for July 6, 1769. Provoked by a murder committed by a lunatic previously considered harmless, the editor wrote: "It is really shocking to see the number of miserable people who have lost the use of their reason, that are daily wandering about, for want of a proper house to keep them confined in. If there had been such a place, this poor man would not have met with the above untimely end." Before 1766, when Governor Fauquier first called for the mental hospital, the *Gazette* seldom mentioned crimes committed by mentally disordered people. After that, and until 1773 when the hospital opened, there were several reports detailing the violence not only of the insane in Virginia but of those in the northern colonies and in London and Paris as well. It is tempting to infer that these accounts were designed to create support for a mental hospital to protect society from the insane.

Unlike the popular American press a half century later, the *Gazette* refrained from describing the insane murderers as beasts or inhuman creatures upon whom society must revenge itself. It reported dramatic cases in a calm, factual manner. For example: A planter who "we hear, has for some Time been disordered in his Mind . . . this Day [after killing his overseer] delivered himself up to Justice, and is now in the publick Jail." A report of a "Melancholy Accident" relates that a wife "long disordered in her senses" struck her husband in the head with an axe and killed him. Another edition of the *Gazette* calls this "a most shocking murder" and describes how the wife broke her husband's skull to pieces by repeated strokes but seemed "quite insensible of the horridness of the crime she [had] committed."

No doubt this noncondemnatory attitude expressed the feeling of at least some upper-class Virginians and made the implementation of Fauquier's proposal easier. That the generally enlightened atmosphere in Williamsburg favored steps to improve the conditions of man, as represented by the hospital, is indicated also by the organization late in 1772 of the Virginian Society for the Promotion of Usefull Knowledge.

Whatever the reasons, on June 4, 1770, a "Bill to make provision for the Support and Maintenance of Ideots, Lunatics, and other Persons of unsound Minds . . ." was received and read the first time in the House of Burgesses. After some debate, though there is no record of what was said, an amended bill became law on the twenty-eighth. The preamble closely followed Fauquier's first message: "WHEREAS several persons of insane and disordered minds have been frequently found wandering in different parts of this colony, and no certain provision having been yet made either towards effecting a cure of those whose cases are not become quite desperate, nor for restraining others who may be dangerous to society. . . ." The governor, councilors, and burgesses of the General Assembly then authorized the construction of a "public hospital, for the reception of such persons as shall, from time to time, according to the rules and orders established by this act, be sent thereto."

[2]

The act gave control of the hospital to a self-perpetuating board or "court of directors." The first board, named in the act, consisted of fifteen laymen: John Blair, William Nelson, Thomas Nelson, Robert Carter, Peyton Randolph, Robert Carter Nicholas, John Randolph, Benjamin Waller, John Blair, Jr., George Wythe, Dudley Digges, Jr., Lewis Burwell, Thomas Nelson, Jr., Thomas Everard, and John Tazewell.

Most of these men bore names prominent in colonial and in revolutionary Virginia. Two later signed the Declaration of Independence: Thomas Nelson, Jr., a merchant who became governor of Virginia in 1781, and George Wythe, member and later clerk of the House of Burgesses, a close friend of Governor Fauquier, and Thomas Jefferson's mentor. Peyton Randolph was king's attorney for Virginia, speaker of the House of Burgesses before the Revolution, and president of the First Continental Congress; his brother John had served also as attorney general. Merchant and planter William Nelson sat on the Council for twenty-seven years and as president of the Council served as acting governor in 1770–1771. John Blair, Jr., was a burgess, clerk to the Council, and later a member of Virginia's first constitutional convention and an associate justice of the United States Supreme Court. Several of the other directors, such as Robert Carter, a councilor, and his kinsman Robert Carter Nicholas, treasurer of the colony, held considerable estates. William Nelson died in 1772 and left the hospital a legacy of £100 for the maintenance of patients, an indication that some directors at least had a personal commitment to the hospital that augured well for its administration.

The board was to choose the keeper, matron, nurses, and guards of the hospital, call in any physicians or surgeons needed, define the duties of employees, determine which patients were to be admitted and which discharged, lay down necessary rules, and generally oversee the hospital's affairs. We do not know whether the General Assembly acted with medical advice in drawing up the founding legislation or whether the first Court of Directors consulted physicians about the organization of the hospital. In any case it would be wrong to assume that no medical knowledge underlay the actions of either the burgesses or the directors (many of whom were burgesses, too), for at that time most educated men knew something about medicine. The wealthy Virginia planter might have a number of medical books in his private library, and he sometimes acted as medical practitioner to his family and slaves on a plantation far away from professional medical aid. Yet, how much the directors actually knew about mental illness or mental institutions is another question. It was probably very little, considering the undeveloped state of psychiatry at the time, the paucity of mental hospitals in Europe, and their virtual nonexistence in America.

Nevertheless, on July 10, 1770, a committee of five—Peyton and John Randolph, Robert Carter Nicholas, John Blair, Jr., and Thomas Everard—set to work to adopt and execute a plan for the hospital. From Thomas Walker they purchased for £112 eight lots of land, about four acres, on the south side of France Street in Williamsburg. To design the building they chose Philadelphia's most successful master builder, Robert Smith, best remembered as the architect of Carpenters' Hall.

Williamsburg was then at a high tide of prosperity. Its small population of nearly two thousand persons (half of them slaves) was augmented during "public times," when the courts were in session, by the several thousand people who crowded its facilities and gave its merchants business. Other large construction projects had been lately completed or were intended. The city and county governments were building a new courthouse (the one still standing); the steeple of Bruton Parish Church was new; and subscriptions were being taken to construct a canal through or near the town to connect Queen's Creek and Archer's Hope Creek.

The main part of town extended east and west for a mile, about half that distance north to south. It consisted of several brick public buildings in spacious settings and some two hundred residences, most of them of frame construction and distinguished by their small outbuildings, yards, fencing, kitchen gardens, and fruit trees. At the western end of Duke of Gloucester Street, the central axis of the town, stood the three buildings of the College of William and Mary, the second college founded in the colonies, chartered in

1693. Some of its Visitors and Governors (as the trustees were called), professors, and graduates were to serve for generations as directors and physicians of the Eastern State Hospital. From the college one could see straight down Duke of Gloucester Street to the Capitol at the eastern terminus. The hospital was to front on France Street about one-quarter of the distance from the college to the Capitol (Figure 1).

Although the original building burned down and the minutes of the Court of Directors relating to the appointment of Smith as architect were lost, his extant drawings and descriptions have enabled a reconstruction to be made of the first plans for the hospital (Figure 2). Smith himself gave a description of the proposed building:

> The Plan consists of a Hall for a Staircase, behind There is the Keepers apartment [22 feet long], and 12 other Rooms chiefly for the Reception of mad People. The Stairs begin near the front Door and lands on passages in the second Story. The second Story has 12 Rooms the same Dimensions as those in in the first Story [each 11′ 9″ by 10′ 9″], and a Room over the Keepers Apartment which may serve the Managers of the Hospital to meet or may be divided which will make two other Rooms for Patients. The Hall is designd to be open as far as the landing of the Stairs the whole hight of both storys. The Cellers shoud be about eight feet high between the under side of the Joices [joists] and the Surface of the Celler floor, And the foundation must go 12 Inches lower which will make the whole hight of the Celler Wall on which you lay the first floor 9 feet. This Wall shou'd be 19 Inches thick either of Stone or very hard Brick and the Partition Walls shoud be 14 Inches thick. The first floor is designed 3 feet above the Surface of the Ground which will require the Wall about 2 feet or a little more raised above the said Surface. This part from the ground up to the top of the first floor shou'd be cased with hard Brick if the Celler Wall be of Stone, unless you go to the Expence of hewn Stone for this part which will be better. After the Wall is worked up as high as the first floor to the full Demensions of the plan set off about 4 Inches for the

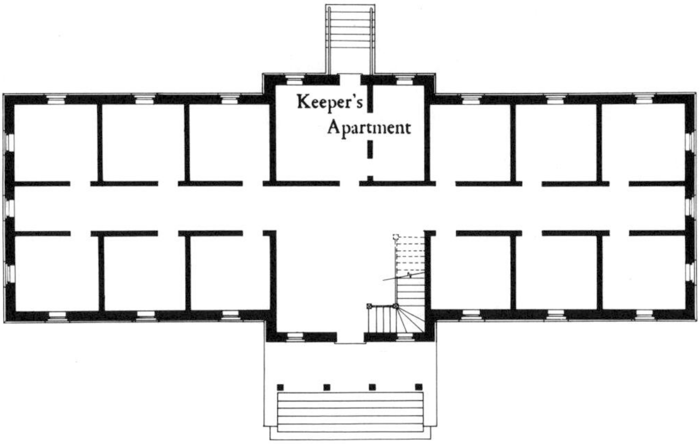

The Public Hospital

Figure 2, above: Ground floor plan by A. Lawrence Kocher and Howard Dearstyne, based on Robert Smith's description and the trustee's agreement with Benjamin Powell.

Figure 3, below: A drawing of the hospital about 1825, possibly later. (Reproduced with permission from *Medicine in Virginia in the Eighteenth Century*, by Wyndham B. Blanton.)

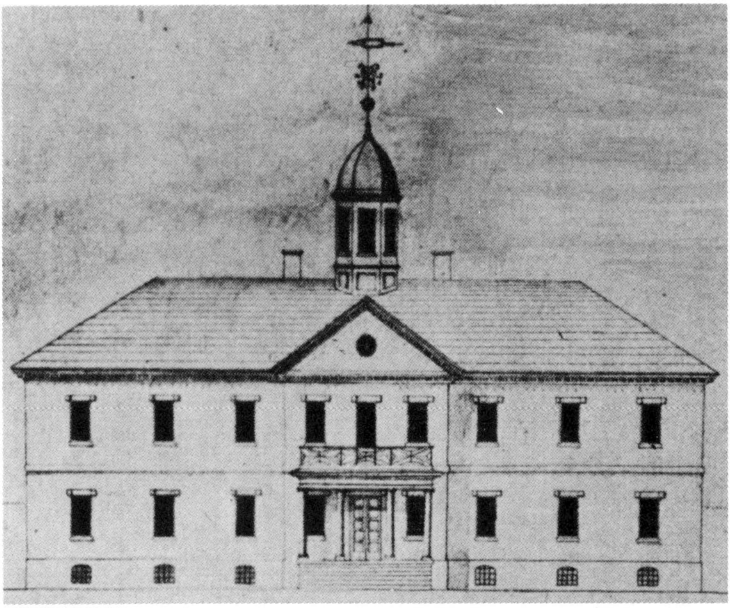

> finishing of the plinth or Water table which may be of Moulding Bricks.
>
> The first Story is ten feet high from floor to Cieling. The outside Walls all round 14 Inches thick and the partitions nine Inches thick of Bricks. The second Story is designed the same thickness and to be Nine feet six Inches high.
>
> The Windows are 6 lights of Glass 10 by 8 Inches for the hight and 3 for the Width, There must be a grate of Iron to the inside of each Window. . . .
>
> If there should be occasion for Fire to warm the common Rooms, there may be Stoves fixed in the Partition between two Rooms with the Mouth open to the Passage, by which means they make fires and the mad People cannot come at them. They shou'd be fixed about two foot above the floor for fear of the Patients falling against the Stoves. . . .
>
> This Building will require about Two hundred thousand Bricks each Brick about 8 3/4 Long 2 3/8 Thick and 4 1/4 Broad. . . . The Bricklayers must order it so that the Chimneys come out in the Roof at Equal distance from the middle otherwise they will have a very ill Effect, . . .

The full dimensions of the building were to be 100 feet by 32 feet 2 inches, the middle section projecting three feet front and back. During construction the directors ordered the thickness of the walls increased by half a brick. Other than iron gratings and padlocks for all windows, devices to prevent escape or to confine patients, such as chains, were not mentioned. The records do not show that the directors ever visited the Pennsylvania Hospital, but Smith's discussion of safety features for patients probably came from a study of that institution. Smith for his part does not seem to have visited Williamsburg, and his advice to construct the cellar of the Eastern State Hospital out of either brick or stone indicates unfamiliarity with humid tidewater Virginia, where stone was not available and even more than brick would "sweat" and make the basement damp and moldy.

From August 2 through October 4, 1770, the building committee advertised in the weekly *Virginia Gazette* that it would entertain bids for the hospital's construction. From September 13 on, the advertisements noted that the plan was at Mr. Jacob Bruce's "for the Inspection of Workmen," and that the committee would meet at the Raleigh Tavern on October 15 "to agree for the Building the Hospital." Benjamin Powell won the contract. He was required to "furnish all the materials . . . except the Grates and such other things as are usually imported from England" and to "compleat the whole in a neat strong and workmanlike manner agreeable to the plan" within two years. The north front of the middle section was to have a "neat Pediment"; the south, east, and west ends were "to be hipped to have a neat Mundelian [modillion] Cornice round the whole—the roof to be covered with plank and good Cypress Shingles." The patients' rooms were to have "strong batten Doors," and good quality wood was specified throughout. The well-burned bricks were probably made near the hospital site, and except for the paint, window glass, window grates, nails and other hardware, and stone steps imported from England, most of the construction material was produced locally.

Work progressed slowly. The directors announced in the *Gazette* that they could not get an agreement for construction for several months and even then the earliest date for which the builder would contract to complete the work was January 18, 1773. The public should not make fruitless applications for admission but wait for a public notice when the hospital would be ready to receive patients. Not only did the construction take longer than the contractor promised, but the original appropriation of £1,200 proved inadequate. The directors petitioned the General Assembly for £800 more to complete the work, explaining that they had at first planned to supply the deficit by subscription but feared it would be improper. They needed £600 for the land and building and £200 to enclose the garden and yards so that patients could safely walk and take the air, to pay a keeper and a matron, and to meet incidental expenses. The assembly granted the request, and work went on until the hospital was finished by the end of summer, 1773.

The plain brick building was much smaller and simpler than either the Pennsylvania Hospital or Bethlehem Hospital in England, despite its being one of the principal buildings of the town and the directors' description of it as "large." In the earliest picture of it that we have, a drawing of about 1825 (Figure 3), the "only touches of architectural ceremony" are the small central pediment, the cornice, and a cupola, but there is no evidence that the original building had a cupola.

The hospital's architectural qualities drew diverse comments. A French soldier in Williamsburg during the Revolution, Chevalier Prudhomme de Bore, thought it a "very fine edifice," as did the famous French traveler La Rochefoucauld-Liancourt; another visitor spoke of a "large handsome brick Mad House (for Lunaticks &c)." Among the less favorable views perhaps the best known was Jefferson's in his *Notes on the State of Virginia*: "The College and Hospital are rude, misshapen piles, which, but that they have roofs, would be taken for brickkilns." A northern traveler, the Reverend Jedidiah Morse, found the hospital "extremely indifferent"; Judge St. George Tucker, a Williamsburg resident defending the town against Morse's criticisms, had to admit that the hospital was among some public buildings that did not seem "to have been constructed with any view to architectural fame." Another traveler was too sensitive to take a good look: "The Mad House is a three Story Building, but as I did not choose to have my Humanity shocked by a Sight of its wretched Inhabitants, I did not go into it."

[3]

Beautiful or not, the building was utilitarian enough, and on September 16 and 23, 1773, the *Gazette* reported the hospital completed and the Court of Directors ready to meet on October 12 to receive patients. The court would meet every Tuesday until further notice, and those sending patients were requested to say whether they could pay all or part of their maintenance; the law permitted the directors to spend the respectable sum of £25 a year for each patient. Restricting admissions to one day a week was common in English hospitals and practical in rural Virginia, where only forty-seven mentally disordered persons were brought to the hospital from 1773 through 1779. Of these, five were returned to their counties as "not proper Objects"; ten were discharged as "restored" to "perfect Senses" (one discharged patient was readmitted twice during this period); five were discharged on security bonds; and ten died in the hospital. Seventeen remained in the hospital at the end of 1779. To get even this small number of patients, financial obstacles had to be minimized. The directors therefore agreed to pay the local sheriffs twenty shillings for the expense of calling together the three justices of the peace who by law had to pass on the insanity of a prospective inmate before he could be sent to Williamsburg. The sheriff was also given five pounds of tobacco for every mile he traveled plus three pounds of tobacco for additional guards if needed to take a patient to the hospital.

Before the reception of patients the Court of Directors had to choose the keeper and a staff. The keeper appointed in September to take charge of the physical plant, the patients, and other staff members, was James Galt; for economy's sake his wife was appointed matron for the female patients. He received a salary of £100 a year plus £25 for his wife. Thus began the service to the hospital by the Galt family that continued for eighty-nine years, a tradition comparable to the better-known association of the Tuke family of Quakers with the York Retreat in England.

James Galt's father, Samuel Galt, a Scotch-Irish goldsmith, emigrated to the New World and settled in Virginia about 1730 or 1735. His large family was prominent in the colony's affairs, especially in Williamsburg, where from 1759 to 1761 he served as keeper of the Public Gaol. Samuel's two sons by his second marriage, James and John Minson, both held hospital posts, and through the next two generations it was their descendants who, with only minor exceptions, held the positions of keeper, matron, visiting physician and then superintendent (Genealogical Table, Figure 4).

James Galt, a goldsmith like his father, was said to have been educated, well traveled, and noted for his integrity and humanity. With his brother, Dr. John Minson Galt, and other leading citizens, he belonged to the Williamsburg Lodge of Freemasons, which he served as junior steward, treasurer, and senior warden. James Galt succeeded his father as keeper of the Public Gaol, a job he kept

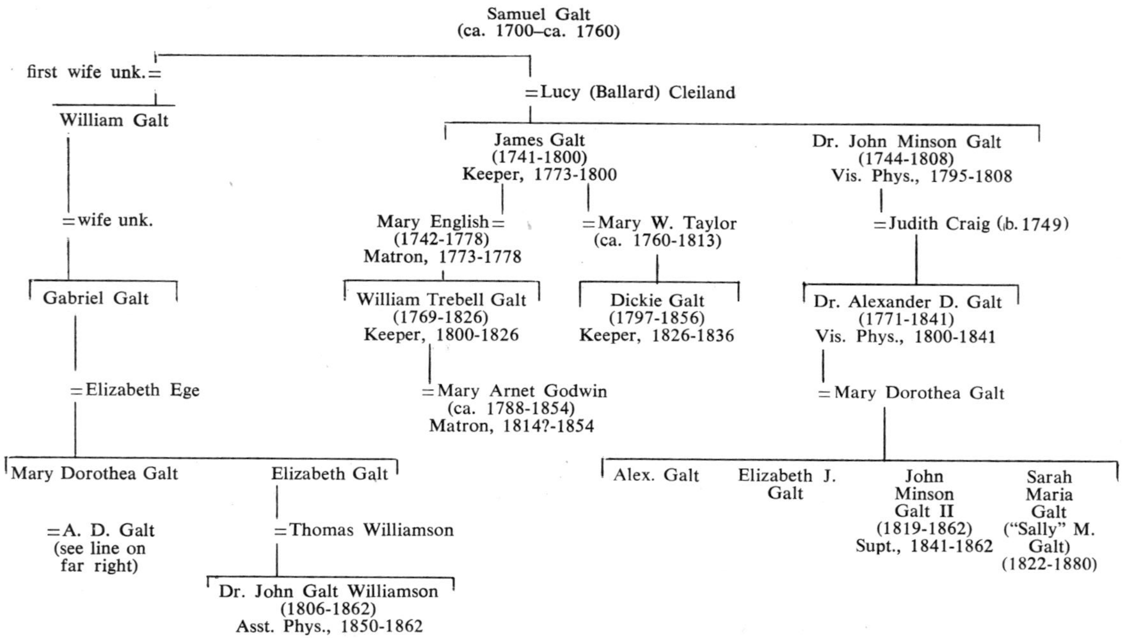

Figure 4

Genealogy of Members of the Galt Family Associated with the Eastern State Hospital

Derived mainly from "Genealogical Chart of the Galt Family," by Rogers Harrison Galt in collaboration with Mary Meares Galt; Virginia Historical Society and Virginia State Library.

until 1766, when he removed to "*Shockoe*, near *Richmond* town" to carry on his jewelry and clock and watchmaking business. Five years later he advertised that on April 1, 1771 he would return to Williamsburg, where he intended to open a similar shop "*on the main Street near the Capitol.*" During the Revolution he was a lieutenant in the Williamsburg militia. He may have, with his family, occupied for a time a small cottage on the hospital grounds (now standing at a different location in Williamsburg but still known as the Galt House). The Galts, along with other local citizens (including some board members), hired out their slaves as servants to the hospital, a common practice until the Civil War.

An attending or visiting physician, Dr. John de Sequeyra (also spelled Siqueyra, Sequiera, and other variants), completed the hospital's staff. It was his duty to see the patients on their "Reception" and then weekly, or more often if necessary.

Almost exactly seven years after Governor Fauquier's original proposal the enterprise was fully launched and ready to receive patients. The hospital was legally open to all "persons"; the act founding it made no mention of slaves. If slaves were accepted as patients it would have been a rare occurrence. The extant records note the commitment of free blacks but not of slaves until the mid-1840s, when special legislation to admit them was passed. Any free person could apply, and if he were admitted the government would pay his upkeep if he could not afford it. Responsibility for hospitalizing the mentally ill was thus placed on the state, a policy then unique in British North America. Despite the hospital directors' protests, justices of the peace seldom described the financial condition of the prospective patients whom they sent to Williamsburg, so that in effect the government of Virginia from the first provided free hospital care for most of the inmates.

Only in 1790 was a fine of £50 imposed for neglect to ascertain ability to pay, but as late as 1831 new legislation on the matter indicated continuing difficulties in collecting information about patients' estates. Ten years later the Virginia auditor of public accounts complained that the law was contradictory and hard to comply with. The governor protested that the state was losing "considerable" sums from "want of means to ensure collections from the estates of lunatics." Moreover, from the beginning the directors of the Virginia asylums, without legal sanction, gave recovered patients a stipend, if they needed it, for clothes and traveling home, a policy that only the greatest financial stringency, during the Revolutionary and Civil Wars, temporarily halted.

[4]

Before the Eastern State Hospital had a chance to establish itself firmly and admit many patients, the Revolution broke out. Less than three years after the hospital opened, the Declaration of Independence was signed at Philadelphia—this only a few days after the adoption in Williamsburg at the end of June 1776 of a new constitution that transformed Virginia into an independent commonwealth. Located in the capital of the rebellious colony and near the coast, the hospital faced physical dangers, and people living at a distance would naturally be apprehensive about transporting their insane friends there during a war. At the same time inflation and shortages of supplies forced a steady deterioration of services within the hospital, so that by 1779 it was probably one of the last places to send a prospective patient.

On October 27, 1778, Keeper James Galt, by then exempt from military service, petitioned the General Assembly for an increase in salary, which had not changed since 1775. In recognition of the general price rise, the House of Delegates (which replaced the House of Burgesses) gave him even more than he had asked for himself and his wife, the matron. The attending physician, Dr. Sequeyra, who had not received a salary since his appointment in 1773, then requested one; he would be willing to accept whatever the legislature thought his services worth. The response was an authorization of £150 for him.

The granting of these pleas showed the good will of the assembly but solved few problems; inflation ate up the increases even before they were received. By June 1779 the hospital's Court of Directors told the House of Delegates that they had deterred James Galt from resigning only by promising him to petition for another increase in the "inconsiderable" salaries authorized for keeper and matron. The loss of an experienced keeper would not only harm the hospital, they pointed out, but it would be difficult to replace Galt at his low salary and it was unlikely that they could fill the then vacant position of matron (Galt's wife had died). Again the House acquiesed, alloting the keeper £200 and matron £100. In October Dr. Sequeyra was allowed, in answer to his request, £250 "for the year past." There was also a shortage of funds to run the hospital, and the directors feared a reduction in the supplies that came to it from the public stores at Williamsburg. Supplies remained short even after the assembly increased the minimum £25 annual support per patient by allowing "a farther sum" of £25 and then again in 1779, £50 each (ostensibly bringing the total sum to £100 each).

Finally the Court of Directors decided that only radical measures would help, especially after the capital moved from Williamsburg to Richmond in 1780. The fourfold increase in appropriations previously voted, they told the assembly in June 1780, did not meet the competition with prices that rose fifty to sixty times—and even more for imported items—so that they had to spend more money than allotted in order to keep the hospital going, a situation they did not relish. Unless they received more support, they declared, they wished to

> disburthen themselves of an Office, which throws upon them the Care of miserable Objects, without the Means of their Relief. Indeed, when they consider the very great Inconvenience which will unavoidably attend the Hospital in Williamsburg now that the Public Treasury and the Board of Auditors are removed to Richmond, they cannot but be of Opinion, that if the General Assembly should determine to keep up the Design, there will be found a Necessity of providing a Hospital at the Seat of Government; as it could have only been upon that Principal, that the Hospital was erected at Williamsburg, so remote from the Centre of the Country.

The assembly did not take this advice; the hospital remained in

Williamsburg. Instead, the Court of Directors was given power to draw clothing and other necessities from the public stores and money from the auditors from time to time as it was needed. Soon afterward British troops began maneuvering in the tidewater area and effectively cut the hospital off from immediate contact with those who could assist it. In July 1781 several directors wrote Governor Thomas Nelson, who had been president of the hospital's Court of Directors, that the hospital was "destitute of every necessary for its support"; that before the British forces arrived the keeper had obtained supplies from the state commissaries through an order from the then Governor Jefferson; that that resource was now gone, and the patients had neither clothes nor provisions. The directors did not doubt that Governor Nelson would do all in his power to help, but in case he could not give the necessary aid and the patients had to be sent home, a list of their names and counties was attached.

Two months later the governor signed a warrant drawn upon the treasurer for £10,000 for the Court of Directors. This apparently large sum was actually quite small, considering the runaway inflation, and possibly sufficed only to prevent the immediate closing of the hospital. The only direct evidence that it may have shut down for a time late in 1781 was a letter by Dr. Sequeyra to the governor: ". . . I must acquaint you, that from the October Session of Assembly in 1769 [1779?] to nov: 1781, the Hospital for Lunaticks being then broke up, I have not received my salary of fifty pound a Year as Physician to the said Hospital, & a hundred pounds is due to me."

Director John Blair wrote the governor on January 4, 1782, that the urgency of the patients' needs dictated violation of the law requiring seven directors as a legal number for conducting hospital affairs. Not able to gather more than five members, the Court of Directors must nevertheless act, for the patients were without clothes and food, the state commissary was no longer at Williamsburg, and the hospital had no credit to buy necessities. The board owed the keeper so much money that he had withdrawn his slave servants and had been only the day before prevailed on to continue in office for a few days. If the Assembly was still sitting, Blair wrote, "Communicate this business to them," otherwise "it would be highly proper to take some measures for returning the poor Wretches to their respective Parishes. . . ."

Blair's letter indicates that the patients had remained in the hospital without interruption, and on January 8, 1782 the state commissaries were ordered to send clothing and provisions to "the unhappy people at the Lunatic Hospital," a further sign that the hospital was then still in operation. Sally M. Galt, granddaughter of Sequeyra's successor, John Minson Galt, and grandniece of James Galt, wrote, sometime after 1862, ". . . during the Revolution, the Institution was used as a Barracks by the Soldiers, & on some of the floors, may be seen where they cut wood. The patients were turned out into the town, & some never returned to the Asylum." This was probably a family story distorted by a hundred years' telling. The Revolutionary armies under Rochambeau and Washington used Williamsburg as a staging area before their attack on Cornwallis at Yorktown in 1781, but that any of their troops lived in the hospital is unsubstantiated. As for the British, they only passed through the town, never stopping for long.

The hospital did close for some four years later on, after the end of hostilities. A new act appropriating the public revenue for the civil government included a salary for the keeper but still left the hospital penniless, as did other legislation. An act to continue and amend the act providing for the support and maintenance of the hospital reiterated the original minimum sum of £25 per patient per annum. Governor Harrison, Nelson's successor, addressing the legislature on October 21, 1782, strongly supported the mayor of Williamsburg in his appeal for funds to save the patients. Nevertheless the hospital remained in desperate straits and finally had to shut down altogether.

Although there seems to be no definite contemporary statement extant to this effect, some evidence supports the suggestion that it closed late in 1782. In January 1784, after the assembly had voted £500 for the hospital in December 1783, the directors wrote the governor concerning payment to Galt, "the late Keeper," of £300, and ordered their president to draw £50 "for the immediate relief of such lunatics as are now in town." When the directors later requested the balance of £150 for James Galt, they did not mention his then being keeper. Galt also received £10 for his "trouble, and expence in saving and securing the paling and other property belonging to the Hospital in the year 1782." A draft for a "Debit of £46.9.8 for the support of two Lunatics at the House of Mr. Galt previous to the reparation of the hospital" presented to the Court of Directors in 1787 indicates that the former keeper remained in Williamsburg and still felt some connection with the hospital; he apparently had taken inmates into his home when the institution was abandoned. The Reverend Francis Asbury, bishop of the Methodist Episcopal Church in New York, who traveled to the "suffering" town of Williamsburg on December 11, 1782, noted in his diary that the Capitol building was going to ruin, the college had but few students, and the "Bedlam-house is desolate, but whether because none are insane, or all are equally mad, it might, perhaps, be difficult to tell."

In 1785 the patient-less hospital was incorporated by act of the legislature, the act to go into effect on January 1, 1787. Before 1785 the legal basis for operation was a series of acts passed from time to time by the House of Burgesses and House of Delegates. In the 1785/86 session for the first time the directors were "constituted a body politic and corporate, to have perpetual continuance." They lost their right of self-perpetuation and would be elected instead, as vacancies occurred, by both houses of the General Assembly; they would from January 1, 1787 be officially known as "the directors of the hospital for the maintenance and cure of persons of unsound minds." An appropriation of £600 enabled the hospital to reopen late in 1786 after completing necessary repairs, including reconstitution of the enclosure as it formerly stood.

Now that they had some money in the bank, the directors decided to appoint a treasurer for the first time, Joseph Hornsby. They rehired James Galt as keeper, his second wife as matron, and Dr. Sequeyra as attending physician. The repairs completed, the directors told the state treasurer that the hospital was in "Condition to receive . . . Patients who have long suffered for want of this humane Asylum." Nevertheless, financial problems remained. The father of one patient was required to pay his son's expenses until the institution received enough money for the purpose, at which time he would be reimbursed. A somewhat similar instance was recorded several days later. At the end of two years, despite the directors' earlier optimism, they again feared the institution must close, because funds voted by the House of Delegates in 1788 had not arrived by the end of October, 1788.

The legislature proved much more able to improve the hospital's position with respect to various legal and administrative matters than to meet its monetary requirements. A law passed on December 25, 1788, provided that the governor instead of the General Assembly would now appoint the directors; their meetings could be held without the presence of their president; and a director moving twenty or more miles distant from Williamsburg automatically vacated his position. The following year the assembly, recognizing that funds for the hospital and other purposes often came too late in the year, passed an act permitting the governor to direct the treasurer of the state to borrow as much money as was deficient out of any other funds and to replace it as soon thereafter as possible.

This last piece of legislation apparently solved no real problems. Continuing unsuccessful efforts to gain adequate financial support finally led James Galt to call on Governor Henry Lee in July 1794, armed with a letter from Robert Andrews, a member of the hospital board, professor at the College of William and Mary, and for a time, secretary to Governor Thomas Nelson. Andrews wrote the governor that he realized that he did not have to apprise him of the hospital's needs and that the governor's orders concerning a draft of money would depend on the state of the public treasury. But he did tell him that the claims on the hospital amounted to nearly the sum being applied for, and he concluded, "I believe Mr. Galt has been obliged to borrow money of his friends for its support."

But where would the money come from? The state government was almost destitute itself: "We have . . . in the public Chest $6,882.97 cents only," the state treasurer wrote, "and we have had for some time past the most pressing demands made on us, on account of the State's subscriptions to the several Canals; the Federal Building; for the support of the Lunatic Hospital, and the public Arsenal, to the amount of more than fifty thousand dollars. . . ."

After an auspicious beginning, then, the Eastern State Hospital had fallen victim, as did other institutions, to the Revolutionary crisis. At a time of financial and political emergency, of physical danger and possible defeat by the British, and then of problems of victory and independence, the government quite understandably tended to neglect the hospital. So did the public. Admission was sought for few patients during these years, and the hospital, small enough to begin with, seemed to share in the general decline of Williamsburg after the capital moved to Richmond.

There may have been popular hostility to the insane or shame about revealing mental illness in one's family, though publication of patients' obituaries and notices of recovery in the *Gazette* and the granting of certificates of sanity to discharged patients indicate an honesty about mental illness unusual at a later time. No doubt Williamsburg's geographical isolation discouraged people from sending patients, as did the large sums granted to sheriffs for the support of insane persons in the county jails. And it would take time for people to be convinced that the hospital sought to cure the mentally disorded of all classes, especially as its directors did little to inform the public of the existence and usefulness of the institution.

When the reopening of the hospital in 1786 brought few patients, the directors did decide to advertise in the newspapers their readiness to receive applicants, but this measure, if carried out, yielded small results. Between November 1, 1786, and October 30, 1790, only thirty-six patients came. Of these, three were removed by friends, eight were discharged presumably as restored, one escaped, nine died, and only fifteen, about half capacity, remained. St. George Tucker observed in 1795 that the hospital never seemed completely filled at any one time, and La Rochefoucauld-Liancourt, visiting Williamsburg in 1796, commented:

> There is besides at Williamsburg an hospital for lunatics, which is supported from the public treasury. It is a fine building; but in it the unfortunate maniacs are rather abandoned to

> their wretched state than subjected to any treatment which might tend to their recovery. From the observations made in Virginia on maniacal complaints, the principal causes assigned for them are enthusiastic devotion and spirituous liquors; and it appears that such as arise from the latter of these causes are less difficult of cure than those which owe their origin to the former. There are only fifteen lunatics of both sexes in this hospital, which is capable of containing thirty.

Another traveler, the youthful Irishman Isaac Weld, badly impressed by Williamsburg in general in 1796, reported that the hospital did "not appear to be well regulated."

The legislature did send a committee to examine the hospital's operation in 1790. The members were appalled at the heavy cost of transporting patients to Williamsburg and sought limits on the number of guards a sheriff could employ for this purpose. They also criticized the directors' negligence in investigating the financial condition of prospective patients so that the ability to pay for their own maintenance could be determined. In the hospital itself, the committee suggested the construction of three cells in the basement for patients in a "raving phrensey" and more privies for the slave servants.

An act to remedy these conditions was passed on December 16, 1790; nevertheless, classification of patients and housing for servants long continued inadequate. Another long-term problem found expression in St. George Tucker's observation that the hospital was "neatly kept, and the patients well attended; but convalescents have not sufficient room for free air, and exercise, without danger of making their escape." The directors took a small step to remedy this deficiency in 1794 when they asked the legislature for money to enclose more land for patients to walk in; but nothing really adequate was done for many years.

Notwithstanding travelers' comments, the Eastern State Hospital's greatest achievement during its early years was to continue to function at all, a feat made possible only by the devotion of the directors and staff, especially the keeper, James Galt. On December 8, 1800, after a quarter of a century at the hospital, he "departed this life," to be succeeded by his son, thirty-one-year-old William T. Galt, at first temporarily and then permanently, at $500 a year. James Galt's second wife, William's stepmother, continued as matron.

Since 1791 James Galt's brother, Dr. John Minson Galt, a surgeon to the Virginia troops during the Revolution and one of Williamsburg's leading citizens, had, together with Dr. Philip Barraud, assisted the aged Dr. Sequeyra in his work as attending physician at the hospital. They succeeded to his job after his death in 1795; Barraud served until 1799, Galt until he died in 1808. The passing of the management of the hospital to the second generation of Galts was then completed with the appointment of John Minson Galt's son and associate, Dr. Alexander Dickie Galt, to his place. The Galt cousins, William and Alexander, served the hospital, as their fathers had, for the rest of their lives. William's second wife, Mary A. Galt, worked with him as matron, probably from 1814, and stayed on after his death until her own in 1854.

[5]

Though the war vitiated their efforts and deprived them of a full complement of patients, keeper and physicians tried as best they could to fulfill the objectives of the founders. Their implementation of these aims, which reflected contemporary medical thought and practice and the enlightened philosophy of the day, was traditional and imitative rather than innovative.

Although recent historical research has rediscovered the existence of therapeutic hospitals in the nineteenth century, the eighteenth has tended to remain within the psychiatric Dark Ages, its institutions usually characterized as custodial. The Eastern State Hospital is a case in point. A standard history of another American mental hospital implies that the Williamsburg hospital was merely custodial: "A small institution without medical organization" or resident physician; a "keeper" was in charge, with a visiting doctor in attendance when patients were admitted or more frequently if necessary. By contrast, the Pennsylvania and New York hospitals were intended for both care and cure of insane patients. Another writer has asserted that "the control of the institution [the Eastern State Hospital] was in the hands of laymen. Commitment, admission, and discharge were not managed by physicians and it is rather doubtful . . . that the visiting doctors had much to do with the treatment of the [*sic*] mental illness." Mid-nineteenth-century asylum superintendents, justly considering themselves pioneers, believed their institutions to be the first therapeutic mental hospitals in the United States.

If the words "without medical organization" mean that physicians neither directed nor controlled the hospital, then the Eastern State Hospital was indeed without such organization—at its founding and for seventy-two years thereafter. Laymen initiated and planned the hospital; a predominantly lay Court of Directors supervised its affairs and decided on admissions and discharges; a keeper, not a physician, ran it from day to day. Physicians probably had more influence in the direction of the Pennsylvania and New York hospitals' psychiatric departments during their early years than they did at the Eastern State Hospital. These were departments of general hospitals, traditionally the province of physicians, and medical men were among their founders. Further, the large and cosmopolitan cities of Philadelphia and New York, in contrast to small, provincial Williamsburg, contained a number of prominent and public-spirited physicians with an interest in mental illness—Benjamin Rush, for example—for hospital boards to choose from and consult with.

If, however, the term "medical organization" implies that a hospital should aim to cure patients through medical treatment applied under the direction of physicians, then the Eastern State Hospital was medically organized from the beginning. Not only was it called a "hospital for the cure of the insane" or of "lunatics," but Fauquier's initial statement envisioned attendance on patients by "able Physicians, to endeavour to restore to them their lost Reason," and the founding act spoke of provision for the "cure of those cases . . . not become quite desperate." Indeed, the Court of Directors tried to exclude untreatable patients. In one case they found the prospective patient harmless, inoffensive, incurable, and therefore inadmissible according to their interpretation of the intent of the act founding the hospital. They sought also to prevent the counties from sending the noninsane indigent, the aged, and the alcoholic—all of whom came to be commonly regarded as candidates for mental institutions.

The directors early explained their position in the *Gazette*. The preample of the act establishing the hospital envisaged admission of only dangerous or curable persons; the legislature did not intend to "exonerate Parishes of the Expenses of their Poor," nor were the intoxicated fit subjects for the hospital. The only criteria for incurability that the directors mentioned were long "Continuance and Inveteracy of their Complaints," whatever that meant. They insisted that the magistrates examining prospective patients take evidence about their condition in writing, because knowledge of the "Causes of the Disorder . . . [might] be of singular Service to the Court, but more especially to the Physician."

In theory, idiots (the congenitally, severely mentally retarded) were eligible for admission, but actually only a few entered the Eastern State Hospital before 1826, when the directors rejected one as not being a legal subject for the hospital; in 1830 they were excluded by law. This policy reflected the belief that idiots never recovered and should not take up space that could more profitably be occupied by a curable insane person.

The visiting physician was deferred to in the medical management of patients—examinations, the prescription of drugs and other remedies, and the like. He also usually participated in decisions about admissions, and his recommendations for discharge were as a rule accepted by the directors. That the latter did not exclude the physician from policy making is further indicated by their appointment of Dr. Sequeyra as a director on January 24, 1774, a few months after the hospital opened. From that time until the law of 1841 required a medical superintendent to head the hospital, the attending physician or physicians usually sat on the court; the attending physician also served as its president from 1822 to 1841.

Control of the operation of the hospital by laymen—the Court of Directors and the keepers—was a common feature of mental institutions, European and American, throughout the eighteenth and early nineteenth centuries. Physicians had as yet neither claimed nor established priority in the field. That insanity was a natural disease, amenable to medical treatment, was accepted in medical circles and among educated people by the mid-eighteenth century; confining total control over the management of the insane to a medical superintendent came much later. Bethlehem had its first medical superintendent in 1853; in private institutions like the Retreat at York, England, founded over twenty years after the Eastern State Hospital, laymen were long in charge; the same was true at the Bicêtre in Paris, where Dr. Philippe Pinel did his famous work during the 1790s. Only in 1841 did the Pennsylvania and New York hospitals give their medical superintendents a significant degree of control over mental patients. That same year the chief medical officer gained formal direction of the Eastern State Hospital. American and British mental institutions established later, in the mid-nineteenth century, were likely to be medically controlled in the modern sense before their older counterparts.

The situation at the Eastern State Hospital, therefore, was not one of conflict between doctor and layman. Both accepted the type of organization there as the best available, based, as it was, on the European model, which Virginians were wont to follow in so many other aspects of their lives. It also permitted physicians to engage in private practice, their service to the hospital being, as in much of Europe, an extension of their function as healers. For it was only during the second decade of the nineteenth century that many physicians specializing in the care of the mentally ill (let alone other doctors and laymen) considered anything but traditional medical measures to be effective therapy.

The day-to-day care of the insane by keeper and matron and the supervision exercised by the hospital boards were not considered invasions of the physicians' province; nor was it an indication that physicians felt hopeless about insanity, as has been suggested. As long as conventional medical remedies composed the primary if not exclusive therapy for insanity it mattered little that laymen rather than physicians had the general management of mental institutions. By caring for the insane in hospitals laymen were seen to protect society and the insane from harm, while physicians would come when needed to attempt to cure patients with physic.

Unimpressive as eighteenth-century medical techniques subsequently appeared to be, most educated people, professional and lay, then considered them the best means of treating mental illness, which was conceived to be a disease of the brain and nervous system that in some unidentifiable way affected the workings of the immaterial mind. No separation, in theory, divided mental illness from other forms of "physical" disorders; all supposedly arose from a set of conditions that varied with the medical system a physician followed.

Whatever its theoretical basis, therapy (especially in England) tended to be heroic: massive doses of various cathartics or emetics, extensive bloodletting and blistering, and prescription of other drugs powerful in their impact on the body though not necessarily on the disease. The impulse to cure mental illness led to the use of these techniques, plus other more specific ones, to the point of inducing debilitation, shock, physical pain, and terror in the patient. Good intent and supposed or hoped-for therapeutic effectiveness justified, as they have frequently done in general medicine, even the most painful and unpleasant remedies.

The system used at the Eastern State Hospital can only be guessed at, especially during the very early years. There is sparse information about the first visiting physician, Dr. Sequeyra, who served from 1773 to his death in 1795. Born in London in 1712, possibly of Portuguese Jewish origin, he studied medicine at Leyden from September 11, 1736, to February 3, 1739, by tradition with the famous clinician Hermann Boerhaave. Since Boerhaave reduced his workload in 1731 and died in 1738, it is likely that Sequeyra also attended lectures given by his substitutes, Jerome David Gaub, who taught chemistry, and Adrianus van Royen, who taught botany.

Unfortunately, Sequeyra left no published record of his medical ideas; nor do extant manuscripts make possible a reconstruction of his system of treating insanity. One cannot even say with assurance that he followed Boerhaave or Gaub. He did favor "natural" (or uncomplicated) forms of medication and moderation in bloodletting, which accorded with Boerhaave's and probably also Gaub's teachings, as did his emphasis on improper digestion in the etiology of illness. We have no evidence, however, to indicate whether Sequeyra took an interest in psychological factors in mental illness, as might be expected if he were a disciple of Gaub.

After Galt and Barraud replaced Sequeyra, the Court of Directors required them to note down the condition of the patients and the treatments given them. From this record book some information can be gleaned about late eighteenth- and early nineteenth-century medical procedures at the hospital.

The "revolution" in psychiatry marked by Pinel's striking off the chains from patients at Bicêtre and the planning of the York Retreat by William Tuke had just begun. Pinel's and Tuke's new system, called moral treatment, de-emphasized traditional medical therapies and regarded the total environment of the hospital as therapeutic; stress was placed on the psychological and emotional state of the patients. The use of shock, terror, and harsh punishment and restraint was modified and eventually partly abandoned. Kindness, consideration, freedom of movement, attention to individual needs and feelings, supervised occupation and recreation, and a family or home atmosphere were all considered vital aspects of treatment and indispensable to the cure as well as the comfort of patients. The physician, whether or not he served also as asylum superintendent, would live on the premises and see each patient daily.

That Galt and Barraud introduced no such innovations, at least on a systematic basis, is not surprising. Through the first quarter of the nineteenth century most American physicians remained ignorant of the new ideas and continued to treat mental patients in the traditional manner. Pinel's classic treatise on insanity did not appear in English translation until 1806, and the first detailed description of the methods used at the York Retreat was published in 1813, five years after John Minson Galt's death. The most influential American doctor of his time, especially among southern medical men, was Benjamin Rush, "the father of American psychiatry," who combined humane and rational treatment of the insane with heavy reliance on phlebotomy, or bloodletting.

Galt, in his day one of the better-trained physicians in Williamsburg, having studied in London and perhaps also in Edinburgh and

Paris, probably knew something of Rush's theories and his practices among the insane at the Pennsylvania Hospital, even though Rush's *Medical Inquiries and Observations upon the Diseases of the Mind* appeared in 1812, after Galt had died. We do not know, however, whether the reforms Rush called for in the care of mental patients and his attention to their psychological state influenced the physicians at the Eastern State Hospital. In only one recorded instance did they recommend to the directors a substantial improvement in the hospital: "a covered Walk within the Brick yards . . . for the protection of the patients from the heat of the Sun." Such a walk was ordered constructed.*

Generally Galt and Barraud seem to have confined themselves to strictly medical remedies; like Sequeyra they concentrated on drugs rather than bloodletting. John Minson Galt loved flowers and spent much time in his garden, where he cultivated the white poppy from which he made opium. He and Barraud also supplied medicines (most of them imported from Europe) to the hospital until Barraud left town for Norfolk in 1799 and ended his association with the hospital. Earlier, when Galt was in partnership with Dr. William Pasteur, he sold drugs to the hospital. After Galt's appointment as visiting physician the directors ordered that instead of buying a medicine chest they would pay Galt and Barraud £10 extra for supplying all the medicines, though family tradition maintains that Galt gave medicines to the hospital as charity.

Galt and Barraud, and then Galt alone, depended heavily on cathartics and emetics, mainly calomel, a form of mercury and one of Rush's prized remedies, and jalap, a botanical. Less frequently used drugs were opium, camphor, vitriol, sassafras, and antimony. It is not clear to what extent medication was prescribed to subdue or punish patients. The cold baths or showers, or both together,

---

* In his general practice John Minson Galt was not "above prescribing English packaged remedies . . . and [publishing] long testimonials of remarkable cures attributed to these patent medicines. . . . Galt advertised Keyser's Pills . . . a cure for nearly every illness. Keyser's amazing 'never-failing' pills, . . . were endorsed by a lord and four dukes, 'performed great Cures in Rheumatism, Asthma, Apoplexy, Palsy, Giddiness of the Head, Dropsey, the Sciatica, or Hip Gout, the Diseases of the Eyes, the Flour Albus, and afforded vast relief in the Gout.'" Harold B. Gill, Jr., "The Apothecary in Colonial America," unpublished research report (Colonial Williamsburg, 1963), pp. 98–99.

that were recorded, sometimes daily for a particular patient, must have been ordered for punishment as well as for therapy and sedation; the occasional warm baths were probably for calming and cleaning patients. What seems evident is that each patient did receive medical care; their number was small enough to allow close contact between them and physicians, keeper, and matron, in contrast to conditions in the large hospitals of Europe.

It is unlikely that the patients suffered from what was then considered harsh treatment. Keeper James Galt's reputation for kindness and the fact that he, rather than ignorant attendants, directly supervised the patients should have protected them against the kind of physical punishment so graphically described in eighteenth-century novels and other writings. His actions were subject to checks through the weekly visits of the directors to give him orders and of the physicians to give medical care. The hospital was so intimate and the town so small that the townspeople would have become quickly aware of any cruelty. We do not know if patients were whipped to control them, as in the Bethlehem and Pennsylvania hospitals, but the records for 1789 and 1790 of a prominent Williamsburg blacksmith indicate that leg irons and chains, another conventional form of restraint, were in use at the Eastern State Hospital.

Further knowledge of how patients fared is sketchy. Except for a few years during the Revolution, they generally had enough to eat, though not always an adequate variety, and were treated with at least a modicum of humanity, even if the personal amenities were meager. In 1787 the directors listed the standard menu, which the physician could change if necessary for the health of an individual inmate—breakfast: water-gruel, mush and molasses or rice, with bread, butter, and salt, or milk; dinner: four days a week, one pound of fresh meat with bread, or half a pound of bacon occasionally, and broth, vegetables, and one quart of small beer each day; the remaining three days: rice, mush, milk-pottage, with molasses or butter, or bread and cheese; supper: any of the foods given at breakfast.

Most patients received the same care, but there was occasionally an attempt to meet the special needs or wants of some patients, especially if they could pay for it. One inmate, the Court of Directors determined in 1790, required "an attention different from that of the other patients in the Hospital," including a private servant, for which he paid a shilling a day. The directors also instructed the keeper to provide him with a "Bed and furniture for one Room" and to furnish him, at the hospital's expense, board from the keeper's "own table." (At that time and for long thereafter the hospital had no "furniture of any other character than that used in poor houses, and other asylums for paupers.") This special patient was shortly discharged because "having been permitted . . . to reside without restraint in a private family [the Galt family] in this City . . . and having uniformly conducted himself in a prudent, rational and peaceable manner, the Court are of opinion that he cannot with propriety be any longer detained here." To the sister of another patient the court allowed a shilling a week because she supplied his breakfast bread.

Generally the Court of Directors operated in a somewhat informal manner. The impression is that it did not always meet as frequently as the hospital's smooth functioning required, a quorum being sometimes difficult to gather. This probably explains how a recovered patient could remain in the hospital for six months before being discharged. Usually "the time of probation," that is, the time needed to convince the physician and directors of a patient's full recovery, was three months during the 1820s and probably less earlier.

[6]

Its conventional methods notwithstanding, the early Eastern State Hospital was in some ways an avant garde, unique institution, though its influence extended not much farther than the borders of Virginia. At the time of the hospital's origin, the immense colony was predominantly agricultural and sparsely populated. It lacked large urban centers where there would tend to be more cases of known insanity, where the insane would be more visible, and where congested living conditions would require the establishment of hospitals for the sick poor, including the mentally ill. But there were unattended cases of insanity in Virginia, some of which had resulted in violence. In Virginians—who prided themselves on their enlightened attitudes (their slave holdings notwithstanding)—the insane seem to have inspired pity and a desire for self-protection rather than hatred or superstitious fear.

Spurred by the British governors, Virginia's colonial leaders stood second only to Benjamin Franklin and other laymen of Philadelphia in making institutional provision for the mentally ill. In so doing they created the first hospital exclusively for the insane in British North America and the first one (the only one for almost fifty years) under government auspices and supported by the state. Its object, however fulfilled, was cure as well as custody, and it was open to all regardless of color, class, or ability to pay (with the apparent exception of slaves). These actions and policies, unusual for their time, set precedents in Virginia and to a small extent elsewhere in the South but not north of the Mason-Dixon Line.

In responding to Governor Fauquier's proposals the Virginian planters and lawyers, living in a society with little fluid capital for privately endowed philanthropic enterprises, seemed to be acting, as Fauquier was, within the old British and continental corporate and governmental approaches to the care of the poor and helpless. And all was done—legislation passed, Court of Directors organized, plans drawn, contract secured, building constructed, and staff appointed—quietly, by a few men, with a minimum of public discussion.

Committees of the House of Burgesses no doubt discussed the matter, but the participants left no known records. The *Virginia Gazette* published only one editorial on the subject and later some brief notices on the progress of the hospital, none of which discussed its character. Royal officials, representing the king, were unaccustomed to courting popular support for their undertakings. They dealt with the General Assembly, a body representative of property holders, many of them well-born, wealthy, educated men greatly involved in public affairs. Anyone of importance in Virginia was likely to serve in the Assembly or be closely associated with it and therefore knowledgeable about its activities and intentions. These were the people who ran things, in government and out of it, an aristocracy that had very much of a free hand most of the time in internal colonial affairs.

Not that the mass of the public would have disapproved such a project as a mental hospital, if only because it would remove potentially dangerous persons from the community. Local residents did not seem to object to having a "madhouse," as it was popularly called, in their midst. It would give the little capital a new source of economic gain, next in importance to the business and employment furnished by political and legal activities and by the college.

In the pacesetting and wealthy northeastern cities, hospital development was different, reflecting the newer model of individual, unofficial action and public discussion. Being privately sponsored, the institutions had to raise funds through popular subscription, which meant that the initiators, acting as private citizens, must educate the public as well as the legislators who would have to sanction a charter and often give subsidies as well. At the same time, though they were nonprofit, the new mental hospitals were designed for middle- and upper-class patients by their middle- and upper-class founders; several were patterned after the York Retreat, with its new system of moral treatment. These included such well-known institutions as the New York Hospital, its psychiatric department founded in 1791 and its Bloomingdale Asylum opened in 1821; the Friends' Asylum at Frankford, Pennsylvania, outside Philadelphia, opened in 1817; McLean Asylum, near Boston, 1819; and the Hartford Retreat of Connecticut (later the Institute of Living), 1824.

The widespread establishment of state mental hospitals came later. Though in the 1820s Kentucky founded a state asylum and Virginia built a second one, the influential and better-known state institutions in the North were not authorized until the 1830s, with Massachusetts in the lead. They were preceded by public hearings, press discussions, publication of pamphlets, and public meetings to convince taxpayers and political leaders of their necessity. The pressure came from middle-class lay reformers imbued with a humanitarianism that saw the community, embodied in government, as having responsibility to redress the social conditions that supposedly caused insanity and other ills.

This movement owed little, if anything, to the Eastern State Hospital. By then Virginia had lost its political and economic leadership in the nation, and communication between North and South, in matters of social reform at least, tended to be one way only, from North to South. The Eastern State Hospital, utilizing as it did slave labor and located in tidewater Virginia, was an integral part of the culture that many northerners, especially reformers, came eventually to scorn.

The hospital had been, moreover, virtually submerged during the Revolution and remained almost unknown well into the nineteenth century; unlike other mental hospitals, it did not publicize itself through articles, books, reports, or traveling keepers and physicians. It also antedated the advent of the moral treatment movement that radically changed attitudes, and eventually psychiatric practices, and stimulated both private and public hospital development. By the time northern states were building their mental institutions the Eastern State Hospital was antiquated and obscure, so that reformers understandably looked elsewhere for inspiration. Like its more ancient counterpart in England, Bethlehem Hospital, the Eastern State Hospital was, in a sense, a pioneer with few known followers.*

* Of the six state hospitals established in the United States before that at Worcester, Massachusetts, opened in 1833, five were in the South. We know that Eastern State Hospital served as a model for one—the Western State Hospital at Staunton. But the scanty published evidence indicates no significant influence upon the others.

CHAPTER II

Stabilization, Stagnation, Reform 1800-1841

[1]

THE Eastern State Hospital, as it greeted a new administration toward the turn of the century, was a small, struggling institution with few patients, removed from the center of power in Virginia, and scarcely known outside the state. It soon developed into a slightly larger but still obscure hospital. In June of 1799 the building was full for the first time, and applicants had to be turned away. Though this was hardly a great feat, considering the small capacity of approximately thirty patients, it signaled a condition that lasted until about 1840: constant pressure to take more inmates than space allowed. The hospital was never overcrowded, however. Unlike later state institutions elsewhere, flooded with patients who shockingly overtaxed the facilities, the Eastern State Hospital accepted only as many as it could accommodate comfortably. The directors sought remedy in expansion of the physical plant, which would also allow separation of the inmates according to their level of excitement. As early as 1804 the legislature authorized construction of an addition. So that sheriffs would not be discouraged from transporting prospective patients who might then be rejected because of the excess demand, laws passed in 1805 and 1807 allowed reimbursement to the "officer and guard" of the expense of returning to their homes persons refused entry into the hospital by the Court of Directors.

If contacts with state legislators or governors were no longer so frequent or intimate as when Williamsburg was the capital, Richmond was not far away, and the Court of Directors knew well at least the local and district representatives to the House of Delegates and the Senate. Much of the time one or another of these gentlemen was also a director. Once conditions stabilized in Virginia, the state government gave the Eastern State Hospital enough consistent support so that serious financial problems did not arise.

The hospital entered a period of stability, especially in comparison with its crisis-to-crisis existence during the revolutionary and postwar years. The War of 1812, in which fighting was not nearly so widespread as during the Revolution, nor inflation hardly so astronomical, seemed barely to affect the Eastern State Hospital, except as the hospital furnished a diversion for soldiers quartered in Williamsburg. (Evidently it was still common for people to walk over to the "Madhouse" to amuse themselves by watching the patients.) Outside of one year, 1813, the hospital's appropriations remained normal and there were no complaints about poverty.

Gathering a quorum (seven members) of the board to admit or reject patients proved difficult, however, and new legislation permitted five directors to perform these functions. Relatively liberal legislative support also meant increased interest in the hospital's affairs, most notably in the form of investigations by committees of the General Assembly concerned about economy, improvement, and systematization of hospital operations. The committees' reports contained recommendations for new legislation and other suggestions that the assembly generally followed.

The first important attempt to regulate the hospital's affairs came in 1822. The General Assembly resolved that the directors should report annually to the assembly, rendering accurate accounts of monies received from the public treasury and from the estates of lunatics and of the disbursement of these funds together with a list of inmates' names, time of their admission, place of residence, and expense of removal. That this requirement came almost fifty years after the hospital's opening reveals the informal relationship that had existed between the hospital and the assembly. As the hospital expanded and state government grew more complex, more formal arrangements and a system of accountability were inevitable.

In 1824 the House of Delegates sent a committee of three to Williamsburg "for the purpose of examining into the condition and wants of the Lunatic Hospital, and the accounts of expenditures of public money for the benefit of the same." They were to report their proceedings and had power to call for persons and papers. The committee found conditions to be satisfactory: all was in good order, cleanliness prevailed, and the gardens and wall surrounding the building seemed in good repair. This impression was typical then and afterwards; the hospital always maintained high standards of cleanliness and sanitation. Sally M. Galt, daughter of Dr. Alexander D. Galt, the attending physician, recalled years later that she repeatedly heard women visitors say it was a model fit to be held up to their house servants. "Indeed, exceeding cleanliness, seemed to be the Genius loci of the place which not even the occupation, by a hostile army, could vanquish or dislodge."

The 1824 committee did find the beds inadequate and the blankets undersized. In its opinion the comfort and safety of the patients required the installation of "close stoves" instead of open fireplaces. The report also disapproved of the custom of paying the matron extra money to make clothes; since she was hired on a yearly basis, the committee argued, all the time and effort she expended for the patients required no further remuneration. In general the committee found the institution "a very expensive one." The cost of meat and wood and of the removal of patients seemed excessive, though members did not know how the price of commodities could be reduced. They did not relate this problem to their observation that the hospital's treasurer was the "principal furnishing merchant," who received a dollar a year for his services as treasurer but made 20 to 25 percent profit on goods sold to the hospital. All supplies were obtained by contract from the lowest bidder, except merchandise purchased for cash.

The investigators paid special attention to the problem of adequate facilities to meet the demand for admissions; "both policy and humanity" forbade crowding the insane together in one hospital. The thirty-five cells for men and thirty for women were not enough; fourteen persons from west of the Blue Ridge Mountains were waiting for vacancies, and their transportation to Williamsburg, some two hundred miles away, would be expensive. To reduce this unnecessary drain on the state treasury and also to provide more accessible facilities for the insane in western Virginia, the committee strongly recommended the establishment of a new centrally located hospital. At the same time the Eastern State Hospital must build more cells for female patients.

The committee reported on the ratio of patients to staff and the cost of maintenance for each patient. In 1823 there were fifty-seven patients cared for by the keeper, the steward, the matron, several other white supervisory personnel, and fourteen Negro slave servants. (Of the latter, eight were male, six female; of them, eight were hired from the keeper, William T. Galt.) This came to about one staff member (including slave attendants) for every three inmates, a high ratio, especially for a state institution treating primarily the lower classes (the wealthy by then could go to the new private institutions opening in the North).

The Eastern State Hospital's unusual advantage of numerically adequate staff—probably accounted for by the availability of cheap slave labor—continued until the Civil War, when many slaves and other staff members left. How many of the staff actually cared directly for patients, that is, acted as "attendants," is not clear; consistent figures are not available, and the number of patients fluctuated greatly from 1823 through the 1830s. Comparisons with northern state hospitals in this respect are especially difficult because of the use of slaves at the Williamsburg hospital to perform various services for patients that white attendants did in the North; these functions, moreover, were not always the same.

The high ratio of total staff to patients at the Eastern State Hospital was likewise an important factor in the cost of patient care. From 1798 to 1810 the average number of patients was twenty-three, supported at an average annual cost of $233 per patient; from 1811 to 1824 the average population rose to thirty-eight, the cost dropping to $186. Costs probably decreased because overhead expenses remained relatively stable while for the first time the hospital's facilities were fully utilized. Included in these figures—and not always in other hospitals'—was the heavy expense of transportation. High prices of commodities, especially in the absence of effective competition for hospital business, were also of significance. During the 1830s and early 1840s, when prices everywhere were higher than in the 1820s, northern state institutions generally estimated each patient's upkeep to be $2.00 to $2.50 a week, or about $110 to $130 a year.

The report of the investigating committee indicated no awareness, either among committee members or the directors, keeper, and physician of the hospital, of the new system of managing the insane—moral treatment on the British model—being introduced in private mental hospitals that opened in the North between 1817 and 1824. In its discussion of the therapeutic accomplishments of the Eastern State Hospital, however, the report did show an acquaintance with at least the statistics of European mental hospitals. The rate of recovery at the Eastern State Hospital from 1798 through 1824 was 38 percent, that is, 135 out of 355 patients were discharged as cured, as compared with an average of 45 percent among the five "best" British hospitals as reported in 1815–1816: "Retreat, Nottingham, Mr. Ricket's, Mr. Bakewell, and the Glasgow Lunatic Asylum." In six other European institutions the average rate was 37 percent, recent cases showing 25 percent more recoveries than old ones. Since many patients came to the Williamsburg hospital after years of confinement in jails and were therefore confirmed lunatics, the committee concluded that the Eastern State Hospital came off well in comparison with the other hospitals.

These figures raise certain questions. The claims of some of the hospitals listed need verification. Even if they are valid, not enough is known about mental hospitals of the period or the kinds of patients they contained to evaluate their recovery rates. Further, the statistical bases were not the same: some figures derived from the numbers discharged, others from the proportion of recent cases restored, and yet others from cures among patients admitted each year. Nor were criteria for cure or restoration uniform, and the number of relapses, if known, would affect curability rates. Nonetheless, at Eastern State Hospital, about which a fair amount is known, there do not seem to have been enough relapses to reduce seriously the reported recovery rates, and, although the directors and physicians left unstated the principles by which they judged sanity, in a rough sort of way it seems likely that most of those they deemed cured were so, at least by the standards of the day.

Thus the hospital, which had changed little since the eighteenth century, managed to restore to sanity about a third of those it treated before 1824. That was a surprising achievement at a time when conventional mental institutions not practicing moral treatment supposedly cured very few patients. Indeed, the Friends' Asylum, one of the first to inaugurate the new regimen in the United States, considered its recovery rate of one-third of admissions during its first two years of operation (1817–1819) to be a marked success. In later years such institutions reported restoring 40 to 50 percent (and occasionally more) of those received each year.

It might also be true that roughly a third of all mental patients ordinarily admitted annually into a hospital—no matter how old or traditional it was—would recover as long as certain minimum conditions prevailed: that the staff considered mental illness curable and attempted to apply therapeutic measures, however antiquated; that patients were treated with some consideration and given a modicum of physical comforts; that the hospital was neither greatly understaffed nor grossly overcrowded; and that not too many patients were chronic.*

As for moral treatment, aside from immeasurably improving patients' daily existence, its contribution may have been to help

---

* Pinel, the asylum reformer, noted that the number of cures at the Charenton asylum during 1798 and 1799 were thirty-three out of ninety-seven patients, "about one third of the whole number; a report agreeing nearly with that of Bethlehem hospital." One should not forget, however, that Bethlehem did not at that time take chronic patients, while Charenton did. It has been observed that the "positive results of treatment obtained towards the midcentury [nineteenth] in the newly built English asylums were attributed by physicians of that time primarily to the ample diet provided." This might have been so in England—though one suspects that more than diet was involved in the matter of mental illness and mental hospi-

restore a significant proportion of a second third of the patients. Only the reappearance of exceedingly pessimistic attitudes, as in the 1880s, saw recovery rates decline below 30 percent in the United States. From about the beginning until the middle of the twentieth century, a period when state hospitals remained generally custodial rather than therapeutic, it seemed that one-third of mental patients ordinarily recovered, another third improved (some enough to return home), and the last third required some form of permanent institutional protection. The Eastern State Hospital, then, with its traditional methods and in comparison with the accomplishments of other hospitals, did fulfill during the early nineteenth century its promise as a therapeutic institution.

[2]

Action followed to remedy the chief weaknesses the 1824 committee found—high cost of operation and insufficient space. The hospital directors justified the large expenditures for supplies by pointing to rising prices, but they acknowledged the need to cut costs in general. The best results, they agreed, would come from having a second hospital for applicants from the region west of the Blue Ridge Mountains, as the committee recommended. To transport one patient from western Virginia to Williamsburg might cost as much as $362.82 in payments to the sheriff and his assistants, the equivalent of more than two years' maintenance per patient.

---

tals—but it was not the case in the United States. At the Eastern State Hospital, in particular, the patients generally ate well throughout, so that diet would not have been an especially significant factor.

My tentative hypothesis explaining the relative success of the Eastern State Hospital during the early nineteenth century is not intended to imply that hospital patients have ever been a uniform mass suffering from a common disorder called mental illness. No doubt mental hospitals have always contained some percentage of nonmental patients (alcoholics in the past and geriatric cases today, for example), and it is probable that the proportion afflicted with certain organic disorders such as paresis has varied. It may be, therefore, that I have compared very dissimilar hospital populations in discussing past results in treating hospitalized patients. Our knowledge of mental illness and its history is too inadequate to do more than speculate. Nevertheless, one cannot but be struck by the claim made over the centuries in institutions with a therapeutic approach that one-third of the patients were restored to sanity. I am inclined to believe that more than chance, or even attempts to create good public relations, has been involved.

On January 22, 1825, the General Assembly agreed to found a new hospital just west of the Blue Ridge at Staunton. The present Western State Hospital opened there in 1828 with a capacity soon afterwards of about thirty-four patients.

Another legislative attempt at economy at the Eastern State Hospital was ineffective: a requirement of 1830 that the hospital must, where practicable, use clothes manufactured at the state penitentiary. The clothes proved so inferior as to be returned on one occasion as unfit to wear.

The space problem was ameliorated but not solved by the new western hospital: accommodations at the Eastern State Hospital had to be enlarged anyway. This was made possible by legislative appropriations sufficient to launch the hospital's first large expansion program. By 1830 it had two new buildings for patients, east and west of the main one, and also, apparently, a new building for convalescents. These additions enabled some segregation of quiet, convalescent patients from noisy, troublesome ones. The commotion at times must have been great; one of his relatives wrote keeper William Galt, "We have no other reason for wishing not to be too near the Mad house but the Cries of the Mad people will increase our Melancholy."

The haphazard administration of the hospital finally stirred the directors to institute some businesslike procedures and administrative order. In 1826 they codified the duties of the keeper. As before, he would compile records of admissions, discharges, and deaths of patients. He also now had to report annually on the hospital property and its condition and on the articles received into the institution, certify all amounts against it, visit patients daily, superintend buildings and their repair, and receive all sealed and other proposals for the sale of goods to the hospital. He was to "exercise a general superintendence over the buildings of the institution, its officers, patients, and servants, and all other things necessary for the good management of the same." To insure the implementation of the new regulations the directors appointed a rotating committee of three of their number to visit the hospital singly or otherwise at least once a month.

Nevertheless, lines of authority remained fragmented and ambiguous. The keeper, in theory given direction over everything but medication, seemed to be transformed in effect into a superintendent. But true centralization of authority over nonmedical affairs was impossible so long as the board retained supervision over the details of administration. Not considering itself merely a policy-making body, with powers to insure the proper execution of its decisions, the board tended to interfere in the everyday affairs of the hospital. The directors treated the keeper like a hired hand—refusing him control over the staff in hiring, firing, salaries, and settling disputes, and encouraging discontented staff members to seek redress over his head. The directors further undermined the keeper's status by expanding the physician's role. The latter was now required to attend the patients daily rather than weekly, which would increase his familiarity with the internal operations of the hospital and perhaps place him at times in conflict with the keeper. An order of the Court of Directors in 1829 prohibited the keeper from permitting "any person to visit patients" without the approval of either the physician or directors; he might also refuse a director admittance if the physician so ordered.

This new rule revealed a broader view of medical treatment and an awareness of the weakness in the existing division of authority between keeper and physician. Medical administration was no longer conceived as synonymous with drug therapy but began to assume responsibilities characteristic of moral treatment—the control of the patients' psychological and environmental experiences. Previously such nonmedical functions had been sufficiently distinguished from medical ones by allotting the latter to the physician and the former to laymen. Now the lines were somewhat blurred. A further complication was the dual role of the incumbent physician: Dr. A. D. Galt was also president of the Court of Directors, and he and the keeper were first cousins.

The establishment of clear lines of authority and definite assignment of responsibility would remain a problem at the Eastern State Hospital for a long time and be complicated by the various family ties among the directors and officers. The tendency toward nepotism was a special difficulty. Other public mental hospitals, while not exempt from it, tended to suffer more from political interference.

The following case, if not typical in intensity and duration, illustrates the kinds of disputes and administrative difficulties that arose. In 1826 William T. Galt, the keeper, died. His wife, Mary A. Galt, remained as matron, and after a few months his half-brother Dickie Galt took the keeper's job. Arguments between Mary Galt and Dickie Galt broke out, she accusing him of unspecified charges and insulting him in an "indecent manner." The directors censured her and placed her on probation for three months; one protested that she should be discharged for destroying the harmony so essential to the proper conduct of a mental institution.

Almost a decade later, the clash again came into the open. Dickie Galt complained that Mrs. Galt was "exceedingly abusive toward him." She charged him, among other things, he said, with appropriating for his own use articles belonging to the hospital. She also warned him that her son would interfere in her behalf, and her son then threatened "in a manner very offensive" to come and chastise the servants. Further, Mrs. Galt frequently employed the servants "in a manner to prevent them from performing their duty," and she spoke against the keeper to patients. She also interfered with his domestic affairs "in a vexatious manner" and lost no opportunity "of vexing and harrassing him."

The directors appointed a committee of investigation whose work was aborted by Dickie Galt's resignation on December 24, 1836. The board then told Mrs. Galt that they did not investigate the charges against her "solely on account of the forebearance of the Keeper, who did not press them." They also "Resolved that the matron be informed that this Board consider the Keeper responsible for all her acts, that She had no independent authority, and that She is bound to obey implicitly, all orders he may give without enquiring into their propriety." While it does not appear that Dickie Galt was actually forced out, the charges he leveled against Mary Galt were such that he probably felt that either she or he must go. The directors evidently did not want to fire Mrs. Galt (the president's cousin by marriage) who had served so long. Dickie Galt may have decided that he had no choice but to resign.

The issue went beyond personal incompatibility or a family dispute. As the directors' statement indicated, it was a fight over authority, one that erupted once again with the keeper appointed to replace Dickie Galt's successor, Henry Edloe, who served only briefly. The new keeper was Philip I. Barziza, the impoverished grandson of a local girl and former grande dame of London and Williamsburg, Lucy Ludwell Paradise, who had died insane in the Eastern State Hospital. Barziza would serve the hospital for years, as keeper until 1841, then as steward, and finally as agent. In 1839 he declared that Mrs. Galt had always sought independent control over the female department "in direct opposition to the express order of this Board." He agreed with Dickie Galt in accusing her of not giving the patients the personal attention common in other institutions and also of causing an "unprovoked and unjustifiable assault upon [himself] by her son, Mr. William T. Galt."

Part of the trouble was that although the keeper had charge of the entire hospital, in the day-to-day care of patients he supervised the males, and the matron, the females. Understandably, then, since she performed many of the duties of the keeper in relation to female patients, the matron sought to exercise the authority of keeper as well. Her position was reinforced by the many years of service without interference that gave her a firm habit of considering the women her special charges. The use of hired slaves for her private benefit was common enough. Other staff members did the same for many years, and most of the slaves belonged to the staff, to the directors, or to the keeper.

Many of these people made money in other ways through their connection with the hospital. Notwithstanding the comments of the investigating committee on the profits made by the treasurer, and their own claim that they generally bought supplies on contract from the lowest bidder, the directors ordered William Galt in 1826 to contract privately or publicly, as he saw fit, for Indian corn. This was preferable to buying corn from the lowest bidder, a practice that had resulted in the hospital being compelled to pay more than the market price, they said. It was better to rely on the discretion of the keeper, who had displayed "zeal, diligence and . . . fidelity in transacting business for the hospital." Later that year Galt's immediate successor as keeper (and Dickie Galt's predecessor), Jesse Cole, resigned after only a few months and on the same day contracted to sell the hospital 250 barrels of corn. Then and thereafter it was common for directors, the treasurer, or the keeper to supply incidental commodities to the hospital and to hire out their slaves as attendants and other workers. Year after year the minutes would show records of these transactions.

[3]

In February 1834 came a revival of legislative discontent over the care of the insane in Virginia. At the beginning of the December 1834 session, and after some controversy over procedure, the House of Delegates authorized a committee to "enquire into the condition and management of the lunatic Hospitals . . . the treatment of patients confined in the . . . hospitals, and in the country jails; the practicability of retrenching the expenses of the maintenance of lunatics, and the expediency of amending the several laws relating to lunatics." The auditor of public accounts was directed to gather the following information: (1) the cost of repairing, enlarging, and insuring the buildings and enclosures of the Eastern State Hospital; (2) salaries of officers, nurses, guards, hired domestics; (3) pay of sheriffs and others conveying lunatics to the hospital and the sums advanced for discharged patients; (4) the amount of miscellaneous expenditures, including the clothing furnished by the penitentiary; (5) cost of confining lunatics in jails and the numbers incarcerated. Similar inquiries were to be made of the Western State Hospital. The committee report on the Eastern State Hospital, issued in 1835, provides a good description of the institution at that time and a thoroughgoing critical review of its operation, along with the directors' and keeper's statements, most of them exhibiting resistance to innovations.

"The buildings," the committee reported, "erected for the accommodation of the hospital, are situated on a lot of four acres of land, in a pleasant part of the city of Williamsburg, to which is attached about two acres of land, on which there is a spring of running water, a bath house in good repair, and a burying ground." The grounds were enclosed partly by paling and partly by a wooden fence, all in need of repair. Except for the washhouse and stable, all the buildings (ten, in 1830) had tin roofs and were of brick. Two new ones were under construction. There were separate yards, enclosed by brick walls to prevent escape, for patients to take the air, and shelters "resting on posts" to protect them from bad weather.

The committee did not note that the hospital had added only two acres to the four it had at the time of its founding, so that its acreage was grossly inadequate by contemporary standards. In the 1840s and 1850s medical superintendents considered fifty acres of land the minimum for an institution capable of housing one hundred patients, which the Eastern State Hospital would be with the completion of its two new buildings. Extensive acreage was supposed to enable patients to engage in farming, then considered a key aspect of therapy. The committee did press for an occupational program that would include the production by male patients of vegetables and dairy items—foods in short supply at the hospital—on some eight to ten acres of rented or purchased land. Such work, plus the sewing of clothes by female patients, seems to have been recommended as much for its assumed economic value as for its therapeutic benefits.

The hospital won commendation as usual for cleanliness of patients and buildings, absence of offensive smells, comfortable conditions, and good general health. The old idea that mental patients, especially violent ones, would be kept under better control if half-starved on a low diet apparently never gained adherents at the Eastern State Hospital. While very few vegetables and dairy products were bought, there was a "liberal" supply of meat, fish, molasses, rice, tea, coffee, and sugar. Indeed, the per capita yearly supply of 440 pounds of meat for 57 patients and 18 hired slaves struck the committee as excessive; slaves in particular, they thought, need not eat so well.

A dining room for convalescent and other well-behaved female patients was needed, the committee suggested. There the keeper and matron, the former living in the hospital, would preside, preserving order and attending to the patients' needs. This proposal—common practice in well-organized mental hospitals of the day—found no favor with the directors, keeper, or matron, who offered the outdated arguments that patients preferred to eat alone in their rooms and that it was dangerous to give them knives and forks. Yet in a few years (by 1838) those patients "capable of appreciating the privilege" were allowed to eat together.

All but a few patients had individual cells in which they were locked at nightfall without heat, with scanty covering, and with no attendants. The committee thought that the slave servants should remain within the buildings after dark to care for the patients, protect them against fires, and prevent escapes. The keeper, however, would not give servants keys to the buildings; nor did he believe it fair to deprive them of time off at night since they received only half the holidays allowed other workers and worked on Sundays as well. As for the servants' living quarters, the investigators found them inadequate and called for improvements, which were subsequently made. The suggestion that more than one patient be assigned to a room met with the objection from the directors that such sharing spread disease. Also damaging to health were the seventeen damp cellar compartments which, the directors explained, therefore remained unoccupied except when absolutely necessary—that is, they would house violent patients, of which the hospital usually had only about eight or ten.

The committee charged that proper classification—the separation of excited patients from convalescents and the grouping of patients with similar temperaments—was inadequate. The directors replied that they did the best they could with their limited facilities, and that the two buildings under construction, with room for about forty more inmates, would improve the situation. The committee noted the large number of seemingly calm patients and questioned keeping them in the hospital. Perhaps they belonged in poorhouses—a suggestion harking back to the idea that the hospital was designed only for the dangerous and curable. The keeper answered that all the calm patients were really insane and not so harmless as they looked. He did not comment about the incurable insane who would be harmless under most conditions and whom the hospital must have included. The directors tried to refuse admittance to such persons, but the law did not permit the discharge of those who became so after entering the hospital.

The hospital's financial records were reported to be in their usual state: a mess. Some of the most important transactions of the board were not recorded, such as the hire of slaves, fourteen from the keeper at $575 a year and four from other persons at $225 a year. The committee did not argue with the prices paid but deplored the irregularity of the bookkeeping. They noted that someone, most often the treasurer, who supplied the hospital with its produce, made high profits: the prices paid for wood, fresh meat, and meal alone rose $500 in one year. "This seems to be a growing evil: where it is to find its maximum, or what is to be the remedy, must depend on the wisdom of the legislature" (which did nothing about it at the time except to require again that clothes be purchased at the state peniteniary). They also wondered whether eighteen slaves were not too many to care for fifty-seven patients. The directors disagreed, but the matron took the opportunity to undermine her enemy, the keeper, by charging that the slaves did not work full time for the hospital; they gave "the residue of their time . . . in rendering services for the keeper."

Possibly influenced by talks with the matron, the committee suggested that she receive a house on the hospital grounds and fuel to heat it, and that she "in an especial manner take all the female patients under her care," clearly something she already did. At the same time the committee disapproved of the directors' practice of dispensing fuel and food to the staff; of their policy of paying the matron for making clothes for patients; and of their view—shared by keeper and matron—that the latter two need not devote their full time to the hospital, but only as much as the patients required.

The full-time presence of the keeper and matron, the committee said, "would soothe the [patients'] excited imagination . . . and a well directed conversation, calculated to draw the mind back from its wanderings, and fix it on things that are rational, (and that often repeated,) might be attended with happy results." Such kind attentions would help the patients to view their keepers as friends, so that the walls of the hospital would no longer appear like those of a gloomy prison but rather a necessary and even pleasant form of restraint. And why were the patients engaged in no amusements? The only reading material found "was a piece of an old Almanac in the hands of one, and the Revised Code in the hands of another." The directors replied that convalescent patients did have all the amusements and books "which the nature of the case will admit." But to the investigators the hospital exhibited "too much the appearance of a well regulated prison, where prisoners are well fed and clothed, and excluded from all rational employment or amusement."

What was more, the reported low recovery rates demonstrated that it had become therapeutically ineffective Taking the years 1833 and 1834 as representative, the committee found the proportion of patients cured to the total hospital population only one in nineteen or about 5 percent. (From 1831 through 1841 this proportion remained on the average below 6 percent.) They mentioned but did not comment on the number of recoveries among patients admitted in each of those years, percentages of 25 and 21, which were also low. A possible explanation for the decline since the 1824 legislative report may be found in a statement by A. D. Galt, made probably during the late 1830s and quoted later by his son:

> The patients now in this institution are generally incurable. They have been under medical treatment, in many instances, either at home or in jails, before they were sent here. It is seldom that a patient is received in the incipient stage of insanity, when the treatment is a very simple process, and when alone a cure can be calculated on with any degree of certainty, unless there be hereditary predisposition.

The directors, however, did not offer such a reply to the committee, which remarked on the uncooperative spirit they encountered: the directors "must have regarded the interrogatory as intrusive, and declined to give such an answer as would have been calculated to have elucidated this interesting subject." Instead they simply denied that the Eastern State Hospital fell behind similar institutions; "if the returns from other hospitals [did] show a larger number of discharges," it indicated "that the cures . . . were not radical . . ." and that therefore many relapses occurred. When asked whether "any further accommodation [was] necessary to promote" recoveries, the directors said no.

Allowing for their tendency to picture the hospital in the best possible light and for the truth of Galt's assertion about the dearth of curable applicants, the impression remains that the directors were more content with the situation than a knowledge of new developments, namely moral treatment, would have warranted. Their attitude, as displayed in their own annual reports as well as in the committee's report, betrayed a continuing ignorance of the new system, which by then had gained acceptance among knowledgeable and interested persons elsewhere and had become established in the new mental hospitals. The investigating committee, in contrast to the one ten years before, did exhibit such awareness and tried to convey it to the hospital's directors and administrators, who seemed sunk in provincialism, habit, and self-interest.

Unlike their counterparts in other institutions—who were reformers, philanthropists, and intellectuals seriously concerned with pathological conditions of individuals and of society and with ways of ameliorating them—the Eastern State Hospital's directors had not kept abreast of psychiatric trends. After the first generation, the board tended to be composed of local worthies with little special interest in mental illness or the mentally ill, though several were men of good will who worked diligently for the hospital. They provided for the basic physical needs of the inmates but neglected the amenities, as well as other innovations that would have made patients' lives more pleasant and less monotonous and confining—labor, recreation, and contact with the outside world, all elements of moral treatment. The adoption of that system might also have helped to raise recovery rates by ushering in a fresh spirit of optimism—as it did elsewhere—so that more patients might be reclassified as curable and would perhaps be cured by the new methods. And only with the changes moral treatment required could the Eastern State Hospital hope to attract recent and presumably curable cases.

[4]

One would have expected that the much respected and intelligent Dr. Alexander D. Galt, also the long-term president of the board, might have shown more modern and sophisticated tendencies and passed them on to the board. But the Galt family's tradition of service to the hospital notwithstanding, A. D. Galt did not seem to be deeply involved in its affairs. His long tenure there, thirty-three years, was characterized by neither strong leadership nor any consuming interest in mental illness, much less in innovations in treatment of the insane.

Like his father, the first John Minson Galt, A. D. Galt had a large private general practice that took up most of his time. His writings, gathered together and published posthumously by his son, scarcely mention mental illness, nor do his extant personal and medical papers. Not that he was unconcerned about the hospital or ignored the patients, whom he was required after 1826 to visit every day. His major interests lay elsewhere, and his self-imposed isolation in Williamsburg, by the early nineteenth century a back-water, no doubt inclined him toward conservatism in medicine and especially in the care of the mentally ill, then still a new and scarcely developed specialty.

He had had an excellent education, though with no special emphasis on mental illness. After graduating from the College of William and Mary, of which his father was a trustee, he went to Oxford from 1792 to 1794 and then to London to study medicine with the well-known surgeon Sir Astley Cooper and observe practice in the wards of Guy's and St. Thomas' hospitals.

By tradition Galt was a talented physician, kind, devoted, and exceedingly modest and generous, whose abilities were hidden away in provincial Williamsburg. A cousin, writing a biography of him after his death, noted, "The distinguished Dr. Philip Syng Physick [of Philadelphia] during the later years of his life in conversation with a gentleman, from Virginia, after enquiring particularly about his old friend [A. D. Galt], remarked 'I have often regretted, that such a man . . . should not have settled in a large City, where the world would have reaped the benefit of his great abilities—Sir he is one of the greatest men in America.' " Dr. Physick, assuming he said something like this, did not exaggerate the limiting nature of life in Williamsburg. An entry in A. D. Galt's diary, when he was about seventy years old, is illustrative. He devoted a section to

"Remarkable events which have happened in Williamsburg & its Vicinity." Included are: August 28, 1841, "Dr. John M. Galt [his son] moved to the Hospital & Slept there for the first time"; and "An account of the Families who have left town this Summer."

The anecdotes about Galt's kindness and generosity, while apocryphal, were probably true in spirit. Despite his extensive private practice his main source of income was the hospital salary. Not much concerned about money, he apparently charged modest fees even to people of means long after his local reputation would have enabled him to do otherwise, and like his father, he was said to have donated all the medicines used at the hospital.

In his medical practice Galt was conventional in depending on depletive remedies, though more moderately than most physicians of his day.

> This, we believe [his son wrote], was the usual practice in the institution from its very commencement: the antiphlogistic [that is, anti-inflammatory] system, together with baths, forming the constituent parts of the medical treatment. Salivation was also restored to in certain cases; and various medicines were used according to the particular indications. In melancholia, he occasionally used tonics. He usually took from eight to sixteen ounces of blood from the arm; this he generally did only once.

Much concerned with the digestive tract and elimination, he would purge with calomel and jalap and prescribe ipecac, antimony, and potassium tartrate as emetics. Though aware of Rush's work Galt seemed more impressed by the eighteenth-century Scottish physician William Cullen, an advocate of less heroic forms of medication.

Galt's view of the proper attitude toward mental patients is presented in his advice to the husband of a woman suffering from postpartum psychosis. "You will find moderate coercion necessary when she tends to do mischief," Galt wrote. "If she attempts to impair her own person you will be compelled to use the strait waistcoat. In your deportment towards her you may be tender, but at the same time you should be uniformly firm & resolute." His papers occasionally mention the restriction of a patient at the hospital to a cell or a strait jacket, or some few cases treated without resorting to calomel and jalap. But discussion of anything other than chemical therapy was rare, so that it can be assumed that patients were, as of old, dosed and purged frequently, albeit "moderately."

Sometimes therapy was given to build up their general health rather than to treat their insanity. This included prescribing small portions of whiskey and rum. The 1832 hospital report notes that "whiskey in considerable quantity, and a small quantity of rum have been used," some for patients, some as a reward for slave servants to clean privies and sewers. The chief use, surprisingly, was for "the cleansing and purifying of . . . patients . . . the necessity frequently occurring of washing the entire . . . patient with whiskey."

It was the keeper, not Dr. Galt, who initiated an extension of the scope of therapy at the hospital in the late 1820s or early 1830s to encompass farming. Including only a few harmless male patients, this practice was not on a scale large enough to please the investigating committee of 1834, nor was it on hospital property. At first such patients worked outside the walled yards at "trifling" jobs; this proved so successful that by 1832 about ten or twelve men began to work on the keeper's farm, which roused community protests that the patients were being exploited.

Not so, said the Court of Directors. The patients considered it a privilege to work on the keeper's farm and regarded withdrawal of the opportunity as a punishment. No work was done in inclement weather or under any detrimental conditions. This program, which aimed initially to improve the patients' physical health, they said, had value also in calming their minds. Although the keeper might earn a few cents, his gains were insignificant compared to the benefits for the patients. Moreover, he gave the hospital many items without charge, such as its full supply of milk. This introduction of farm work seems to have occurred independently at the Eastern State Hospital, unrelated to psychiatric practice elsewhere.

Far removed from the new hospitals (and probably never having visited them) and more deeply immersed in general medical practice than in psychiatric problems, A. D. Galt remained committed to the traditional medical treatment of mental illness and to an uncompromisingly somatic view of it. His allegiance was much stronger than that of most young reforming medical superintendents, including his counterpart at the Western State Hospital, Dr. Francis T. Stribling. The question of whether mental illness is a "physical" or "mental" disease, though perhaps a false one, is ancient and still unresolved. The point is not who was right, but that in retaining a virtually complete reliance on physical remedies, Galt remained out of the mainstream of the thought of his day on mental illness and its treatment.

During his last years, when many measures characteristic of moral treatment were introduced at the hospital in the aftermath of the 1835 legislative committee report, Galt still resorted chiefly if not entirely to medication, as some of his case histories show. He summarized in his diary the ideas of a contemporary French author who stressed the medical aspects of patient care and also a British physician's prescription for curing melancholy: one gram acetate of morphia every evening and a dose of castor oil every other morning for some weeks. Galt was also impressed by the Frenchman's use of long immersion of patients in tepid baths.

In 1839 he made two copies of the sixth annual report of the new Worcester (Massachusetts) State Hospital, which had the reputation of being the leading public mental institution in the United States. Its reports, compiled for educational as well as official purposes, circulated in editions of three thousand copies and contained extensive accounts of moral treatment as an auxiliary to traditional medical therapeutics. The section of the report that Galt stressed maintained that mental illness was "generally . . . one of the most curable of diseases" if treated before becoming chronic, that is, within a year of onset. This was a particularly relevant point for the Eastern State Hospital, with its many already chronic patients.

It is possible that had the hospital not come to contain so many incurables, Galt might have been inclined to initiate or at least discuss the innovations that seemed to be having success in the North and in Europe. It was, however, not likely. By the late 1830s he was sick and old and sharing his medical supervision with the keeper in order to have time for his private patients. Bringing the

Williamsburg hospital up to date with modern practices would have to come, as it did, largely through outside initiative and be enforced by a new, young superintendent. Galt tacitly admitted as much in composing in 1841 a letter, apparently never sent, resigning his position at the hospital.

During most of its second major period, then—the first forty years of the nineteenth century—corresponding more or less to the regimes of Alexander D. Galt, the physician, and William T. Galt and Dickie Galt, the keepers, the Eastern State Hospital was always expanding and, though not allowed to become overcrowded, never lacked for patients. It was able to obtain sufficient support from the state and to furnish various citizens of Williamsburg with lucrative sources of income. The patients, though not mistreated, lived a pallid and confined existence. The quality of life offered them had not risen much above the stagnation that afflicted Williamsburg. Like the town, the hospital was somnolent, small, antiquated, and dull.

[5]

Williamsburg was passive but Richmond would force it into action. The critical conclusions of the legislative investigating committee in 1835 produced no immediate results, but in conjunction with other forces they eventually led to improvements designed to lift the hospital from the eighteenth to the mid-nineteenth century.

A significant sign of change was reported by the influential Prison Discipline Society of Boston, interested in the mentally ill because so many of them still lay in prisons. The society reported that the two lunatic asylums in Virginia had each received in 1838 the large sum of about $30,000 from the legislature and that the superintendents had been visiting similar institutions for purposes of learning how to improve their own. (The so-called superintendent of the Eastern State Hospital was Philip Barziza, the keeper.) The next year the society again reported the activities of both the Eastern and Western State hospitals and in so doing perpetuated the incorrect idea that they "were both originally designed for pauper lunatics, and such have generally been accommodated." That "many patients of other classes" were sent to northern institutions was true; that only pauper lunatics went to the Virginia state hospitals was not. Unlike most state hospitals founded later elsewhere, they took in all classes, rich and poor.

The Western State Hospital had been opened in 1828 as a traditional institution in which conditions were not much better than in the Eastern State Hospital, though it had a good deal more land. Striking changes came after 1836 with the arrival of the new attending physician, Dr. Stribling, twenty-six years old, enthusiastic, well-respected, and determined to improve the hospital. A trip north immediately after his appointment stimulated him to transform the Western State Hospital into a modern institution whose innovations were to enlighten the governor of Virginia about the marvels of moral treatment.

By 1842 the Prison Discipline Society listed Western State among asylums that had attained a high degree of excellence. They were

> without exception, beautifully located. They are all supplied with good gardens; most of them, with many acres of fertile and cultivated land; a considerable number, with large and productive farms. They are constructed of good materials,—stone or brick,—on the general plan of a centre building with wings. They are under the superintendence of very superior men. . . . The assistant physicians, stewards, matrons, and attendants, have been chosen with great care, and are, many of them, the very salt of the earth. The principles of government and conduct are religious and Christian to an admirable degree. The employments, recreations, amusements, instructions, and influences, are very various, and well fitted to soothe the excited, cheer the desponding, guide the erring, check the vicious, raise the fallen, and restore the insane. The restraints are very few.

As for the Eastern State Hospital, it sent no information and published no annual reports. This was unfortunate, the society implied, as such reports were the "one thing more calculated to promote the improvement and usefulness of an Insane Asylum" than any other.

The directors of the Eastern State Hospital were beginning to realize that their institution resembled only slightly the model described by the society. They gave indications of wanting reforms, no doubt influenced by Barziza's findings up North and more especially by pressure from the legislature and the governor. Their 1839 report virtually admitted as much: "The recent enlargements of the establishment, and the liberal spirit manifested by the general assembly, have made it the duty of the board to revise its regulations, and to endeavour to adopt such changes as might make the success of the institution commensurate with the reasonable expectations of the public."

Early in 1837, after Dickie Galt resigned, the keeper was required to give full-time service to the hospital, and the directors received permission to spend up to $1,000 for, among other things, a "neat two horse carriage," a pair of horses, and land for a garden. The introduction of "modern improvements," the directors said in their 1838 report, would be possible if the Assembly approved the construction of a new building so that the patients would have more physical comforts and moral treatment could be employed. The directors supported changes introduced by the keeper:

> Thus, dress of a character somewhat superior to that ordinarily allowed, has been given to those capable of being influenced by it: cheap musical instruments . . . to some who know how to use them—also the means of playing at various simple games—solitary meals have given place to an assembling at a table of those capable of appreciating the privilege, occasional attendance at church, and excursions into the neighborhood . . . for . . . relieving the tedium and monotony of confinement, and soothing or amusing the over excited or wandering intellect.

An order promulgated after Barziza returned required him to purchase materials to enable patients who were mechanics to "employ themselves in such a manner as may be beneficial to their health and the interests of the institution." The board intended, it warned the legislature, to use further devices to restore patients to sanity even if an increase in expenditures was necessary. That all the changes it described as already in force could be accomplished without larger appropriations indicated either previous padding of the budget or the limited nature of the new program. The directors' self-righteousness seems peculiar in the light of their having, just the year before, elected one of themselves keeper at the same time as the salary for the position was raised two hundred dollars, over the protests of two directors. This keeper, Henry Edloe, served only a few months.

At the end of 1839 came perhaps the strongest push for change, a statement from the governor, David Campbell, in his annual message to the General Assembly. During the summer, he had visited the Western State Hospital, accompanied by the physician, "whose untiring efforts to improve its usefulness are worthy of the highest commendation." He observed "the order and neatness which pervaded the whole establishment, and the comfort of its inmates [and] was especially gratified to learn the number of the insane persons that had within the last year or two been cured and discharged, to return again to their homes." It was too bad, therefore, that the present hospitals in Virginia had not enough room for all the insane in the state and that their friends did not take them to the hospitals as soon as they became ill, when they had the best prospects for cure. Three days after the governor's message the House of Delegates appointed a committee to determine a method to increase the capacity of the state's mental hospitals.

Governor Campbell's successor, Thomas W. Gilmer, visited both the Eastern and Western State hospitals, arriving in May 1840 at the former, where he "was engaged two hours in making inquiries relative to the management of the Patients, then planned improvements in the new buildings & observed that he did not wonder at the few discharges, the patients being paupers & incurables, &c, &c." Reporting to the House of Delegates, Gilmer regretted that so many of the insane were still in jails, to the great expense of the state and to the detriment of their condition. The two asylums he found in good order and well managed, and he acknowledged the gratitude due their physicians and directors "for the assiduous attention and improved methods of treatment" they were introducing.

With such encouragement and pressure the directors of the Eastern State Hospital broadened the practice of moral treatment. Their 1839 report pointedly noted that for the past six months "not even a mitten, much less a strait waistcoat, has been required. A gentle rebuke or a few hours confinement to the room has always been sufficient to recall the power of self control." As part of their new program, the directors drew up a questionnaire for persons committing patients, in order to help direct treatment in each individual case. The board felt that the public should be informed as to why the hospital appeared to be so far behind others, in Virginia and elsewhere, "in effecting what should be the main end of all lunatic asylums"—cures. "The reason why so few have been cured . . . is that we have not received for years, what may be termed a recent case." The various improvements in and expansions of the physical plant, in process and planned, were calculated to widen the activities and amusements of patients, especially the curable ones, and also to enable the admission of more patients, whose illness, they hoped, would be recent and therefore more amenable to cure. The board tried, unsuccessfully, to give preference to such applicants, for whom twenty-one cells were set aside.

A serious hindrance to their efforts and an explanation of their plight, the board considered, was the discrepancy in admissions policy between their hospital and the Western State Hospital. Under existing law the Blue Ridge Mountains formed a boundary line for the regions from which each hospital would draw patients, but prospective patients could apply to the other hospital if refused admittance to the one in their zone. The Williamsburg board had understood the law to require the admission of patients in order of application, regardless of extent of illness. At Staunton, the directors interpreted the law (as had the early Court of Directors of the Eastern State Hospital) to permit refusal of long-standing cases in favor of recent ones. The rejects would then come to the Eastern State Hospital, its directors complained, and thus reduce the places available for recently stricken applicants and help keep recovery rates low. The Eastern State Hospital was thereby in danger of being converted into "a hospital of incurables." The legislature might then hold back funds for so ineffective an institution, and curable patients would avoid it; what purpose, therefore, in introducing improvements designed to cure patients?

Understandably, the directors requested a law prohibiting either asylum from accepting patients "from a county nearer to the other asylum than to it, so long as there may be upon the register applications from counties nearer to the latter than the former." Such legislation was necessary to protect the Eastern State Hospital's reputation as a therapeutic institution. Even before then the Eastern State Hospital had requested Western State Hospital to take all applicants from its zone and save the state the transportation money east; after all, the Western State Hospital had been founded partly on that account.

It was perhaps in response to this plea that the House of Delegates resolved on December 11, 1840, to instruct its committee on lunatic asylums "to enquire into the report to this house, why . . . the number of patients cured in the Western Lunatic Asylum so far [exceeded] that of the asylum at *Williamsburg*." The report referred to was probably that made by a committee appointed December 2, 1840. The delegates also expressed concern about the treatment of patients: on December 10 the House inquired whether the practice of the ducking stool or any corporal punishment was continued in either of the Virginia state mental hospitals. If so, could not some "mode of discipline and punishment less terrific and severe" replace it?

The legislative culmination of the reform movement in Virginia came on March 6, 1841, when the General Assembly revised the existing laws relative to lunatic asylums. A significant feature was the abolition of the boundary line for applicants to the two institutions: the new law provided that patients had to apply first to the nearest one; if they were refused, the other, if it had room, had to take them. Another important directive was that the boards of both the Eastern and Western State hospitals "appoint a superintendent (who shall in all cases be a physician)."

This measure finally ended the dichotomy of leadership at the hospitals and brought them into conformity with administrative practice at the best new contemporary mental institutions. Actually Stribling had become superintendent of the Staunton hospital some months before, when the directors reorganized that hospital on the plan in effect at the asylum at Worcester; they then called upon the legislature to require a physician to head the mental hospitals of the state. At Williamsburg the directors responded to the new regulations by resolving on April 24, 1841, that "The Present Surgeon Shall act as Supt. & the present keeper as steward, & . . . all other officers Shall continue in office, at present Salaries, till same Shall be suspended." The "Present Surgeon," Dr. Alexander D. Galt, was seventy years old and so ill that he had not been able to work for months and would not live long. He expected his son, John Minson Galt II, just finishing his medical studies, to succeed him, as indeed soon afterward he did.

CHAPTER III

Modern Treatment: The Psychiatric System of John Minson Galt II 1841-1862

[1]

WITH the accession of John Minson Galt II the Eastern State Hospital continued to move into the modern era. If Galt was by his youth and personality perhaps not the best man for the superintendency, he did, through his professional activities and intellectual abilities, lead the hospital into the company of similar institutions in the United States. Through his sensitivity and kindness he gave new and intimate attention to the needs of the patients. Not so isolated from the medical and psychiatric world at large as his father, and required by law to confine his medical practice to the hospital, he was forced, at first reluctantly and then with enthusiasm, to dedicate his professional efforts to psychiatry, to which he made some useful contributions.

Nevertheless, the hospital continued to suffer from a certain provincialism, and many old problems persisted, exacerbated by John Minson Galt's temperament and inclinations as well as by the mere fact of his appointment. Some indication of the power of tradition and of the low status of the superintendency of the hospital can be seen in the fact that the position was given to a twenty-two-year old youth just out of medical school. He probably had had no training at all there in psychiatry, a subject scarcely touched on in medical education after Benjamin Rush's death in 1813, but he would have had contact since childhood with patients from the hospital. Though there were probably other applicants for the superintendency, tradition and propinquity won out, and now the third generation of Galts began to serve the hospital.

The third child and second son of A. D. Galt (the first son was consumptive and died as a young man), John Minson Galt II was talented, precocious, and much doted on by an adoring and protective mother and two neurotic, sickly maiden sisters. He was sheltered and secluded in his domestic circle and educated as a child by his mother, a "woman of high intellectual endowments, & refined literary taste." Though much absorbed in books and study, he was also in his youth something of an athlete. He attended the preparatory school down the street at the College of William and Mary and, like his father and grandfather, entered the college; there he read the classics and wrote articles for the *Southern Literary Messenger.*

After graduating at the age of nineteen, he studied with his father for a time and then went to the Medical College of the University of Pennsylvania in Philadelphia, from which he graduated in the spring of 1841. His dissertation concerned the family hobby that he shared: botany. Much to his mother's and sisters' regret, he planned to stay in Philadelphia for a while longer to learn the "practical part of medicine . . . such as drawing teeth & mixing medicines." "I never drew a tooth or bled any body in my life," he confessed, "and it is a great deal better for me to learn these her[e] than to have them to learn when I come home." He soon returned to Williamsburg to take care of his father and work as assistant physician at the Eastern State Hospital, where he took notes on its management from Barziza, the keeper, and "Aunt [Mary] Galt," the matron.

Everyone except himself expected John Minson Galt to take the superintendency and felt sure he would do well. A gentle, scholarly person with little administrative ability and not much self-confidence, he felt "quite disgusted at going to the Hosp." but hoped he was becoming more accustomed to it. At the same time he was upset about an apparent delay in receiving the office his dying father so much wanted him to have. Never one to praise his children or express his feelings, A. D. Galt extolled the care given him in his last illness by his son: "No physician ever prescribed with more skill. John will be a blessing to the Institution over which he presides, & an Ornament to the World." Others of the Galt clan predicted great success for the young man. He studied hard and was "voracious" in his intellectual appetite, though he did suffer from dyspepsia, "that curse of the studious," and did not take "sufficient exercise in the open air." Only his older sister Elizabeth later expressed doubts. She feared he would founder on "the *rock* on which our whole *generation* split, viz. the want of *proper confidence*."

John Minson Galt II noted this quality in himself. In the diary that he kept during much of his adult life, he wrote in 1841, "I should endeavor to succeed by reading in insanity—for in this I will rise above all although I fail in other things." While still in medical school he confided a fear that he was unloved, unrespected, and disliked; women did not consider him manly, though he felt he could make himself agreeable to them.

> I put these things down . . . from the desire . . . to correct an idea which is perpetually seizing me that those around think me inferior to them, do not care for my company, & therefore . . . I [am] often led to be rude, and indeed to reject the advances & treat . . . badly some who like me. . . . My own reserve & solitariness increase this. Somehow I have lately taken a pleasure & a pride in increasing this solitariness. Indeed the pleasure of this pride has often led me to sit silent an[d] alone when I might have done better. My conduct has thus sometimes amounted almost to rudeness even to ladies. I must endeavor to conquer this at least for the sake of having good

> feelings instead of these improper ones of pride & too much independence. . . .

These confessions may seem to be the perhaps irrelevant secret thoughts and ambivalencies of any normal young man with a tendency to introspection. In John Minson Galt II, however, they revealed problems that were to remain with him all his life and help to keep him in Williamsburg, unmarried, constantly worrying about his health and complaining of anxiety, fond of company but much wrapped up in his books and his rigorous, self-imposed plans of study, yearning for fame but remaining comparatively obscure and somewhat aloof from the small, intimate group of asylum superintendents of which he could easily have become an active part.

Despite his fear of failure and his inexperience Galt believed he had no choice but to work at the hospital, to which he finally became "almost wholly reconciled." Though he looked "with some dread to practicing," he contemplated "with much pleasure . . . the little pleasures attending every family circle—the newspapers—gossiping &c," and "with eagerness . . . [to] the ball on Monday night." Would his "expectations of pleasure be realized?" He was appointed superintendent on June 1, 1841, as of July 1. His father, after suffering for nearly three years from "almost every Disease which man is afflicted with" died calmly the following November 20. The "funeral procession was very large every body was anxious to see the last of the *good man*," and the Court of Directors of the hospital composed an eloquent eulogy to his "unpretending worth."

Once in office, John Minson Galt II sought distinction in his new profession through publication of his writings. With some notable exceptions most American asylum superintendents of that time excelled in administration and medical practice; they were primarily executives and practitioners. Galt was of a less practical and more intellectual and inquiring nature, which he well realized. To attain fame "with regard to insanity," he wrote, "I should be cosmopolite perhaps, notwithstanding the scattered character of our population & the small number of our asylums. Hence study & making myself known by observation & writing." He observed that "the affairs at the Hospital are of long-waiting—What have I then à faire que à étude [*sic*]."

During his first year at the asylum he ordered from England what his father's library lacked, standard contemporary works on insanity. He put himself on a strict schedule of study and contemplation, with many injunctions on duty, self-discipline, and self-denial, and much guilt over his lapses. His diary is replete with comments on how his illness interfered with study and on his struggles with anxiety. Much concerned with religion, he also had an excessive portion of the gloom and self-agonizing so often found among "delicate" nineteenth-century youths. "O agony" reads one diary entry; others tell of blue, disconsolate moments.

With all his problems Galt produced a fairly large number of articles, including two series of *Essays on Asylums for Persons of Unsound Mind*, initially given as reports to the Association of Medical Superintendents of American Institutions for the Insane, of which he was one of the founders in 1844. His annual reports, first published for the year 1843, also served as a vehicle for his ideas, and he occasionally wrote for the *American Journal of Insanity*, begun in 1844 as the first American psychiatric journal, the precursor of the *American Journal of Psychiatry*. The youngest of the pre-Civil War generation of American psychiatrists, Galt was the widest read (he claimed to have the best library on mental illness in the United States) and the most scholarly. He was also the most versatile linguist: it is clear that he knew French, German, Italian, Greek, and Latin. From notes taken from European monographs on insanity he published a book of excerpts in English, *The Treatment of Insanity*, a real service to a new profession with a sparse literature and members untutored in foreign languages.

Wide-ranging in his intellectual interests, Galt wrote several articles on politics, including strong pleas for the annexation of Texas. He liked to think of himself as a Jeffersonian democrat, but in regard to the crucial questions of the day he was actually a conservative, pro-slavery, states-rights, southern expansionist who usually preferred Whig candidates and attempted to reconcile Jefferson's concepts of equal rights with Calhoun's doctrines.

Retaining his fondness for literature, especially the Greek and Roman classics, he continued to read widely and published critical essays on poetry, as well as on botany and other scientific subjects.

It was in his psychiatric writings that Galt displayed the originality and flexibility of thought that were to place him among the few asylum superintendents of his day who distinguished themselves through contributions to the psychiatric literature. Characteristically their best work did not fit the contemporary model of systematic "scientific" investigation in psychiatry—the correlation of post-mortem studies, usually of the brain, with symptoms of mental illness.

Galt did suggest a procedure that, if adopted, would have facilitated pathological studies, but he was not himself interested in pathological research and did little of it. In view of the popular aversion to autopsies and the difficulty in a rural state of communicating with the next of kin of deceased patients, he proposed making legal inquiry of relatives at the time of admission whether they would allow an autopsy in case the patient died. He also participated in the widespread practice of uncritically compiling statistics on supposed causes of insanity; his reports contain, for example, superficially analyzed figures relating admissions and discharges to seasonal changes. But this was a minor endeavor. Like his other intellectually oriented colleagues, Galt relied mainly on observation, intuition, and logic in his explorations of psychiatric problems. His were scholarly studies, summaries of his wide reading, and descriptions and analyses of his experiences and observations.

Methods to test objectively the claims of physicians, especially psychiatrists, were then at best in embryo. There was as yet no national climate of scientific research in medicine or psychiatry. Certainly none existed in backwater Virginia, where as late as the 1850s manifestations of a flourishing and organized medical profession—an effective state medical society, substantial general hospitals, medical journals, outstanding medical schools—were either weak or lacking. Galt, isolated in Williamsburg, had to depend mainly upon his library, travel, correspondence, and clinical experience.

[2]

For all his timidity, youth, and intellectuality, Galt did seriously tackle his job as superintendent, and with characteristic thoughtfulness and determination. He would do his best to learn about mental illness and modernize the hospital's organization and administration, which meant, basically, to introduce a full-blown moral treatment. Unlike the attending physicians before him, he was required to devote full time to the hospital, to accept no other compensation, and to treat no private patients. He had under his supervision the "general government of the Asylum and all its appurtenances; . . . the direction and control of all the patients, and of every person employed in or about the Institution, subject to the rules and regulations of the Court of Directors." When requested he must attend the meetings of the court as well as "prepare and put up all medicines which require his attention." He would not, however, have the full command usually granted the chiefs of corporate mental hospitals and a few chiefs of state institutions, among them Stribling at the Western State Hospital. For example, the directors, by law, still admitted and discharged patients, with the advice of the medical superintendent. More significantly, control of hiring and firing personnel and determining wages remained with the Court of Directors, thus perpetuating the danger that political considerations or nepotism would influence appointments. The directors also continued to take a rather close interest in the hospital's day-to-day affairs.

Still, for the first time the hospital had a chief, a talented and intelligent physician concerned solely with its administration and devoted to applying the best in contemporary medical thought to the care of his patients. Theoretically in charge of most of the operations of the hospital, he could consolidate medical and nonmedical treatment, that is, all that might contribute, through a controlled environment, to the cure of insanity. His responsibility as a physician, therefore, went beyond traditional prescription of drugs, baths, and diets, to the administration of occupational therapy, recreation, exercise, and restraint, and to the conscious creation of an atmosphere of kindness and benevolence. This removed from the keeper, now named steward, much of his former sphere of authority, though he and the matron could still be the primary executants of the new policies, so much of them being nonmedical. There was always the possibility that these lay supervisors could in actuality control a major part of the life of the patients if the superintendent did not maintain firm direction.

At the outset John Minson Galt II effected an improvement in the tone of the Eastern State Hospital. Following the advice of the famous phrenologist Johann Spurzheim that the physician utilize his own personality in his therapeutics, Galt decided to concentrate on "mildness & firmness," which he considered his forte. His "mildness" was immediately felt. In 1842 a visitor who knew the hospital well spoke of the great change for the better; in the past it had been "merely a sort of jail." Others also wrote of the good Galt accomplished and of his close interest in the patients.

In 1843, two years after his appointment, the young Galt went to Philadelphia to see about publishing his father's writings and took the opportunity to tour mental institutions, a common practice of new asylum chiefs, some of whom visited Europe, too. From what Galt learned on his inspection of nine hospitals and from his extensive reading, he developed a set of ideas about insanity and its treatment that greatly influenced patient care at the hospital. They were for the most part conventional theories and practices among American physicians specializing in mental illness and among educated laymen concerned with the mentally ill.

Some of his emphases bore the impress of his own personality and thought, as well as unique circumstances at the Eastern State Hospital, though his more original ideas were implemented only imperfectly or not at all. Because the hospital was comparatively small (only 109 patients as of July 1, 1841, with a capacity for 125 to 130) and the need for reforms well recognized, Galt was given a rather free hand to experiment with schemes that did not involve heavy expenditures. A discussion of his ideas, as related to practice, can therefore give a picture of patient care under his administration, particularly during the 1840s, the main period of innovation.

Galt accepted the general theory that the insane differed from the sane in degree of deviant behavior and thought rather than in kind, a view that justified in his mind treating the insane as nearly as possible like normal people. Where the thin dividing line lay must be determined in each case with reference to the history of the patient and his total personality. Galt did classify the varieties of insanity as "many delusions, few delusions, weakness of intellect, morbid feelings," all of them stages of a single disorder that had as its basis some physical morbidity. As to exactly what morbid condition insanity depended on, he wrote, "we have as yet perhaps not an entire agreement; though it is viewed by the mass of physicians as depending on some morbid states of the brain." He agreed that there were two main types of causes, predisposing and exciting, that somehow acted upon the brain and hence the mind to produce insanity. Predisposing causes—physical or social conditions difficult if not impossible to control—served as necessary preconditions, or inflammatory material, as it were; exciting causes—temporary but potent forces more amenable to manipulation—set off the conflagration.

Experience convinced him, however, of the difficulty of determining causation in particular cases and of the inadequacy of relying on simplistic lists of causes often derived from sparse information furnished by patients' relatives. He early recognized that the causes of insanity might frequently remain hidden, to be revealed perhaps by carefully questioning those who accompanied patients to the hospital "as to every fact which they know." More significantly, he brought to bear his own experience with

> secret sorrows . . . treasured up and brooded over in the lonely heart. Things, seemingly of little consequence, are felt by some persons much more than they deserve, and far more than others imagine. . . . With the sane, too, as well as the insane, imaginary evils sometimes cause as great or greater distress than real ones; for instance, we look forward with dread to events which are imaginary; never occurring, at least in the shape which we had previously given them. Such secret causes may insanity have.

The search for hidden springs of madness led Galt to stress multiple, psychological-physical causation and encouraged an emphasis in therapy away from his father's almost total reliance on medication. At the same time the popular theory (as influenced by phrenological ideas of brain function) that the brain was divided into several faculties seemed to dictate measures designed to occupy and thereby strengthen the brain so that "its morbid ideas and feelings shall become inactive, and be thus gradually enfeebled or effaced."

There was a theoretical obstacle to the use of psychological methods. Physicians adhered to a somatic view of mental illness, not only because of their traditional commitment to somaticism and its attendant somatic therapies, but also to convince laymen that insanity was a natural and treatable disease rather than an incurable, shameful calamity. But if insanity was ultimately a physical disorder that somehow manifested itself in a deranged mind, and if mind and body were separate entities, how could psychological measures affect the disease? This contradiction was not satisfactorily solved and mid-nineteenth-century psychiatrists relied instead on experience as a guide.

So with Galt. At first he reported that "generally medical means [were] chiefly applicable to recent, and moral means to chronic insanity," that is, medicine could effect cures and moral treatment could improve the living conditions of incurables. A few years later he was applying moral treatment "more or less to every case," though he continued to insist on the undoubted value of medication. By 1853 he was less sanguine about the latter's role in therapy, a change reflecting the experience that patients who received no medication sometimes recovered. Then he saw no difference in the rates of cure in hospitals using a vast variety of medication but all agreeing as to the efficacy of moral measures. "Must not the deduction be plainly adverse to the utility of medical means to a very great extent?" Like so many psychiatrists then and later, Galt assumed that if patients recovered they did so because of some therapeutic measure employed at the hospital, so that if medicines were not responsible, moral treatment was.

He did not completely give up traditional treatment but applied it more sparingly than before and mainly to relieve symptoms rather than from any faith in its curative value. A maniacal or violent patient, particularly when first admitted, could not, he believed, benefit immediately from moral therapy but had to be placed in an unfurnished room, dosed with narcotics, and, if still unable to control himself, given shower baths or restrained by wrist bands or mittens. Of most benefit were narcotics, tonics, purgatives, and counterirritants. Galt tested some of the newest drugs suggested by European medical men and found them wanting.

In his own remedies, though, he had considerable confidence. Opium he regarded as the best narcotic; he used it in the form of salts or morphia, mixing them with tobacco for smoking or in brandy for internal use. (Smoking was allowed freely at the hospital until 1859, and its prohibition afterwards seemed to produce no visible effects on the patients.) The doses were large, because Galt believed that "*all* insane persons are perhaps less affected by opiates than the sane, except the cases of idiosyncracy." Among other things, opium removed a symptom of insanity, insomnia, and in so doing acted "morally, by withdrawing the mind from its delusions." And in a drugged state the patient might be persuaded to work. In later years he spoke favorably of the local "Thoroughwort plant" (a species of Eupatorium) as an effective tonic.

Another tonic frequently given was sulfate of quinine, especially in cases of debility; salt of morphia was added if excitement was present. With all his modernity Galt showed himself a true son of his father and conventional physician in his belief that there were few cases where purgatives did not prove useful. These commonly included neutral salts, mercurial preparations, castor oil, croton oil, aloes, and tincture of hellebore, all administered, except for the mercurials, every other day; mercurials, twice weekly. Counterirritants he found most valuable in cases of torpor and for patients passing from an acute to a chronic state; the agent was the common blistering-plaster, applied to the back of the neck.

In print Galt always either opposed bloodletting or recommended great moderation; it had never been popular at the hospital and by 1850 had been abandoned by many leading mental hospitals and was falling into disrepute even in general medicine. He wrote privately, though, that he considered it in theory proper as a sedative at the beginning of an attack of mania. The most "marked benefit in subduing nervous irritability and excitement" came, Galt observed, from warm baths—the French system of "irrigation"—continued for one or two hours or longer, while cold water was sprinkled "gently" on the head, and from showers in the morning and warm baths in the evening. He thought much more use could be made of baths as a therapeutic measure in acholism.

Galt's original contributions at the hospital were nonmedical, that is, the various measures associated with moral treatment. He saw two great principles involved in this system, the substitution of kindness for harsh means and the replacement of isolation by efforts to "act on the morbid faculties revulsively, by calling other and undiseased faculties into exercise."

As for the first, only kindness tended "fully to dispel the vague ideas, often present in the insane, that those around them are their enemies." The confidence thus inspired made possible all manner of treatment and led the insane, even when violent, to vent their anger in fantasies rather than against the staff. By kindness he also meant close attention to the patients' symptoms and needs, not for days and weeks but for months and sometimes years, including attempts, through questioning, to discover patients' feelings and thoughts. "We judge from the information so acquired that we cannot determine always the mental state by the outward manifestation." Perhaps by a "careful investigation of this subject, a classification might be made of these concealed states of mind, and thus a new resource be given to aid us in determining what course of treatment was certainly indicated."

In several cases he found that patients were afraid of the people with whom they came into contact. Consequently he realized the futility and indeed provocative tendency of using harsh means to eliminate the violence arising from such fears. Further, certain ridiculous actions performed by the insane "may be only a giving way to feelings which we all have and like homicidal madness would follow from weakened mind." From these investigations Galt did not evolve a systematic explanation of the thought processes he studied, and his recognition that the illogicality of the insane would vanish once their motives were understood was not new. But even to try to discover these hidden feelings and motives and apply them in therapy was unusual at that time.

The other great principle of moral treatment, reduction of the patients' isolation, was effected, Galt said, by the endeavor to make their situation similar to that of the sane in as many ways as possible. But then why take patients out of their homes in the first place? Because they sometimes recovered in a hospital, seldom at home. Hospitalization did not mean total removal from the sane world and sane people. It was an attempt to substitute healthy influences for the morbid associations at home and to provide the skilled care and protection not always obtainable from relatives and friends. In this process everything and everyone in the hospital influenced the patients, contributed to restoring the curable, and made life more pleasant for the incurable. Most important was continuous contact with sane persons, both to offset the injurious effects of patients on each other and to help them overcome their delusions and impulses.

In the spring of 1843, shortly after Galt returned from his tour to the North where he saw the principles of moral treatment in practice, the board approved a plan of organization that would help him to create such a therapeutic environment. This included patient classification. Galt separated patients first by sex and then into four major classes: the quiet and calm and convalescent; the violent; the demented; and a group that worked outdoors. Further division would be impractical in a small hospital, he thought, but should any class of patients contain enough persons with similar characteristics another subdivision would be warranted. Patients kept together in small homogenous groups would become accustomed to each other and came to share points of view, developments which were beneficial to them and which helped them to pull each other out of their reveries.

The different groups were placed in various wings of the hospital, whose appearance Galt considered therapeutically significant: a hospital must provide more than just a minimum of physical necessities in a gloomy conglomeration of buildings. He suggested, for example, refurbishing the porticoes of the center building and extending them to the wings, and painting the whole exterior, which on account of its having been erected at various times presented a "motley appearance." Then and later he stressed that this could affect patients particularly when they first arrived, distrustful and apprehensive of torture, their minds converting dilapidated hospital facilities into places of horror: thus their worst fears were confirmed. The "impressions of the insane mind on entering an asylum, are sometimes of the utmost consequence; on their nature may depend the event of the case, whether the patient shall henceforth be lost in the darkness of insanity, or shall regain the light of a rational mind."

The chief feature of Galt's reorganization involved developing a staff of high quality, something the Eastern State Hospital lacked in comparison with northern institutions, where complaints on this score were also common. Intelligent and dedicated staff members, assigned only to serve the patients and given specific tasks in relation to them, would be concerned with their rehabilitation rather than merely their safekeeping. Several would be craftsmen, such as shoemaker, tailor, and carpenter, who doubled as attendants and occupational therapists. In the North, Galt said, attendants slept at the hospital and sat up with the patients in the evenings, so that patients did not have to retire at dark.

As he expressed it later, these various attendants, called officers, were to "soothe the insane mind on the one hand, and on the other to draw forth its torpid faculties into exercise, and to restore it to a healthy activity." They were, in a sense, the administrators, nurses, occupational therapists, and attendants of today's hospitals, and Galt, like hospital reformers of the mid-twentieth century, tried to draw all of them directly into the therapeutic process. This would give the hospital "a class whose self-respect as officers or quasi officers, will raise them above the mere servants who act as attendants in other asylums"; they could be recruited from a "good class of Society," as in the exclusive McLean Asylum in Boston.

Here is Galt's scheme as it worked out:

> . . . the male department is divided into four sections, over each of which sections an officer is placed, termed in the by-laws attendants. These officers see that the servants [the hired slaves] behave well toward the patients, and keep their wards in order; they attend too to the wants of the patients,

> and seek to engage them in different modes of occupation and amusement. Moreover under charge of one of these officials is the shoe-shop in the Gothic building, and the tailor's shop is under care of another. There are likewise two attendants or officers, who walk out with the patients, assist the ward officers just spoken of . . . and have besides, that which is of the most extreme importance, the special supervision of certain lunatics, who would otherwise be almost necessarily under restraint or in seclusion—the reduction of restraint and seclusion to a minimum being a [illegible word] in the progress of Asylums.
>
> Like the male department, the female department is placed under four female attendants or officers, who have similar duties as to the female patients and servants, to those fulfilled by the analogous functionaries on the other side of the house. They have besides, the task of employing the insane inmates daily in sewing, . . . with the aid of the Tailor's shop, to make up all the clothing worn by the State patients.

Two of the male groups stayed outside the wards the greater part of the day and therefore required only one attendant. Those remaining indoors were cared for by an officer and a servant. This arrangement resulted in a striking change over the past, Galt said. Patients previously unmanageable were now easily handled.

After years of experience with the system Galt felt positive that it resulted in a "greater degree of uniform kindness to our insane inmates than exists in any other asylum elsewhere." He felt continuously able to trust every one of the officers as implicitly in this respect as if he were present at all times. How successful he really was is difficult to know. Detailed information about the way the staff actually treated patients is not extant, and Galt's contemporaries might have had a different conception of kindness and a proper staff. Dorothea Dix, the great crusader for better care of the insane, criticized the Eastern State Hospital in 1848 for having too few competent, intelligent attendants and nurses and too strict a tone, showing "traces of the old system."

In any case, whatever Galt could accomplish in this regard depended a good deal on Negro slavery. Slaves hired out to the hospital did all the menial work, serving as orderlies, cooks, and launderers, and in some cases as attendants. It was thereby easier to engage a "better class" of white personnel and give them a higher status than attendants in northern hospitals. Indeed, Galt boasted that the Eastern State Hospital could carry out the injunction of kindness on account of just this advantage.

He did acknowledge certain drawbacks in the use of slave labor in a progressive hospital. If moral treatment required careful classification of patients and intelligent, devoted companions for them, then, it was believed, slaves could not be used as attendants. Galt shared the prejudices of his colleagues in thinking that only middle-class whites should supervise white patients and could have the proper moral influence upon them. But white persons to take care of the difficult group of demented white inmates were hard to find, so he had to put Negro slave servants in charge of them; this was not so terrible, he concluded, since the minds of the demented were so weakened and irredeemable that a black attendant would do.

Another disadvantage of employing slaves was the patients' isolation and neglect at night because the hospital management feared to trust slaves with the keys. (Night guards were not appointed until March 1854, one male and one female.) Further, patients would not help in the kitchen and laundry because slaves worked there. True, middle- and upper-class patients sometimes refused to work simply because they considered such activity beneath them under any circumstances. But there is no reason to think that the stigma the southern slave system gave to manual labor failed to affect southerners even when they were insane.

A possible objection to female slave servants was implied in an entry in Galt's medical diary: "I told [a director] to oblige me by not mentioning my name in connection with that of [a servant], first because I never had anything to do with any woman hired by the Hospital, and secondly no Gentleman would have anything to do with a parcel of women who either let the male patients have intercourse with them, or acted as to cause such a report." What justification Galt had for his charge is unknown. He did not mention slave women having "improper" relations with patients except this one time, when he himself was implicated.

It was not easy to eliminate slave labor at the hospital. When one director sought to reduce the number of slave servants, another resisted because he did not want whites doing the menial duties. Presumably, too, those hiring out slaves to the hospital would also be opposed. And though slaves were "objectionable," Galt complained, ". . . they could not be dispensed with, as white servants were not procurable." The steward suggested, to no effect, hiring eight Irishwomen to replace the slaves, on the assumption, probably, that they would do the same work for not much more money at a time when labor by Irish immigrants was valued in quality as well as in cash as little above that of slave labor.

The slaves continued to work at the hospital until the Civil War came to Williamsburg. Galt never denied that some worked well; a few he praised highly, and he employed one recovered free black patient to care for the black male patients. At one time he unsuccessfully opposed the dismissal of the best and most experienced women slaves, who cost the hospital extra money by keeping their children with them. Even slave labor was at a premium. To insure the employment of satisfactory servants the hospital early in the 1840s adopted Galt's proposal to pay 15 percent above the market price to their owners, and Galt offered to attend sick servants free of charge. Nevertheless a competent slave labor force was never assured.

[3]

As much as he could, Galt tried to create for the white patients a family feeling, to give each one similar accommodations to those he had at home while sane, provided those were comfortable, and a daily life essentially unchanged. After the first paroxysms of violence, fear, and withdrawal, a new patient would be introduced into a social situation, first within the hospital and then in the community. If all went well, he would move from less to more privileged status. After leaving the isolation of his room, he would eat with other patients and eventually with members of the other sex at the table of the matron or steward. He might then have the freedom of the hospital grounds, go on supervised excursions into the neighborhood and, before 1851, even walk unattended into town. By this time he would probably be engaged in some form of labor and various sports and games and might visit Galt's home at will. There patients "were ever welcome guests & almost daily partook of his hospitality."

> They may be said to have constituted an element in his domestic circle, & they were thus withdrawn as much as possible, from their morbid delusions by the agreeable realities surrounding them. A library, pictures, & works of art, natural curiosities from foreign lands, together with his ever agreeable conversation & explanations of what they saw, were used with great success in soothing the agitated feelings, rousing the torpid intellect and helping to restore the darkened mind. . . .

Galt "was almost adored by his patients," according to one biographical sketch, whose author declared that the visitor to the hospital

> . . . was filled with heartfelt gratification & admiration, to behold the affection with which these unfortunate people regarded their beloved physician & friend. He would walk among them in his daily rounds, addressing each one, with the greatest respect & listening to their absurd remarks, with as much gravity & respect, as if they had been the utterances of the greatest philosophers. He would converse with them earnestly upon any subject upon which they were able to talk rationally, & it was his constant endeavor, to strengthen any slight glimmerings of reason, that might be elicited, & by every means to make them satisfied with their condition.

His sisters came to know many patients well. When Sally Galt went to Richmond, Elizabeth wrote how much several of their insane friends missed her, and after Galt's death a former patient lived with Sally for years. Dr. John Galt Williamson, Galt's cousin and closest friend and later his assistant at the hospital, "frequently spent an hour or two in playing draughts with the patients."

In his attempt to surround the insane with a normal environment, Galt rejected the old, no-longer-popular psychiatric idea that patients must be denied contact with outsiders. He welcomed visitors to the hospital, where they broke the daily monotony. One year he reported having ladies from Williamsburg come:

> If an arrangement could be made by which a few of them would visit the institution at stated times, various beneficial consequences would result to the patients. . . . Doubtless in the dim perspective of life's journey, which the children of affliction are here pursuing, such visits would be truly as bright stars.

In later years complaints about too many visitors led to proposals to limit them by requiring passes; traditionally the boys from the College of William and Mary came freely to the hospital for the amusement of watching the patients. Galt objected that restrictions would eliminate most visitors except relatives, the only group he specifically did not want inundating the hospital: ". . . otherwise I did not care how many persons saw the patients." The public also might assume that the hospital sought to hide something, to which a director replied that the public complained of the reverse. Galt lost, and on October 11, 1854, the gates were closed; the next day the first permit for visitation privileges was issued.

Occasionally a special visitor would create a pleasant stir. When Dorothea Dix came to Williamsburg on her periodic tours through mental hospitals around the country she quickly established affectionate relations with the Galt family, the patients, and the staff, including the servants. She was interested in and concerned for everyone and seldom came empy-handed. On one trip she brought books, pictures, and "fragments of Ribbon & Mousseline, to convert into bed-quilts & fancy work." From merchants in New York and Philadelphia she wangled "books of patterns of ribbons, silks &c sent from Paris" to distribute among various asylums. She also sent a group of pictures for the servants and patients. One picture was given to a blind woman because "it would give her so much pleasure to show to her friends," Sally Galt wrote to Miss Dix. It meant "so much for her to have to say that a Lady so many miles off should think of her." The pictures for the inmates were divided equally between the men's and women's quarters, "to be kept a month in each ward, & showed on rainy days to the Patients; so that they will seem to them as new, for a long time."

Various amusements, aside from their value in occupying patients, seemed to Galt therapeutically useful in breaking into the patients' self-concern and encouraging social intercourse among them. He did not try to supply all possible forms of amusement, as he had learned from experience that patients would choose what pleased them, that different groups would prefer different kinds, and that preferences would depend in part on the patients' mental condition. Generally he found that they liked the same pursuits as did sane people and that convalescents especially would play games much as if they were completely sane: ". . . in amusement as in other matters, the policy seems best, to treat the insane as though they were sane; and moreover, not as children, but as men and women." In 1843 he was authorized to buy books, periodicals, and musical instruments.

Galt has been called a pioneer in music therapy in American mental hospitals. Actually, the directors of the Eastern State Hospital had the keeper buy instruments for patients in 1838, before Galt came. In his belief that music drew the mind from delusions and morbid emotions Galt may have extended this policy, but if he achieved any first in the United States it was probably in calling attention to this effect through publishing a passage from Shelley's "Julian and Maddalo" describing the benefits of music to inmates of a Venetian madhouse. We do not know just how much he encouraged musical performances at the hospital, but a Senate investigating committee in 1845 noted that music was "cultivated and much practised." There are only a few references elsewhere to concerts for patients; on one occasion patients played the piano for Miss Dix.

Galt's contribution to bibliotherapy has also been discussed in an article indicating that his views, while enlightened, were unexceptional. As more middle-class patients came to the hospital he found that some who would not readily engage in labor did enjoy reading.

The hospital had for a long time furnished some books and newspapers to patients who wished to read, and in 1840 it had subscribed to a newspaper and journal. These had served merely to assuage the patients' voluntary desire for reading, not "any strictly curative purpose."

Galt thought there was need for a regular library, and that it "would be worthy of investigation to observe what effect certain books have had upon [the] ins[ane] and how." In 1850 he wanted to try an experiment of systematic reading as opposed to desultory reading; since formal education proved far superior to occasional reading for sane persons, it might have equally good effects on the insane. Except for "reading and voluntary study or composition, we possess no immediate mode of acting on the intellectual powers, resulting from a regular effort on the part of some person" working at the hospital. He favored classes, discussion groups, lectures, or some combination of these.

He did succeed in setting up what the Senate investigating committe called a "small library." After complaining that the hospital received no donations of books and newspapers, he finally expressed thanks in 1847 to editors for supplying newspapers free of charge; in 1853 he suggested the expenditure of one hundred dollars for the library.

His patients' library was no innovation. The Friends' Asylum at Frankford, Pennsylvania, for example, had begun a library and museum in 1838 as part of its extensive system of moral treatment. Where Galt did pioneer was in being the first to write formally and at length about bibliotherapy in his "On Reading, Recreation, and Amusements for the Insane," first delivered in 1848 as a talk before the Association of Medical Superintendents and later published as one of his *Essays on Asylums for Persons of Unsound Mind* (Second Series). He also supported the idea that mental hospitals should accumulate libraries on "psychical subjects" for the use of physicians, including annual reports of other mental hospitals.

As for formal educational programs, in 1854 the directors ordered Barziza, then the hospital's general agent and supervisor of the gasworks, to act as a teacher for the patients if his other duties permitted. At the same time they authorized the employment of a female night guard who would also teach classes for women patients during the day at the discretion of the superintendent. It is not clear whether these "teachers" ever actually held classes. In 1859 the hospital announced for the first time a series of "Lectures as a Means of Treatment." Who gave them and how frequently was not said, but an unpublished biographical sketch of Galt notes that he lectured to the patients on such subjects as "Painting & Painters," "Theology of the Floral Kingdom," "Conversation," "Aurora," "Nephele or Glimpses in Cloud-land," and "Music." The Pennsylvania Hospital had begun such programs in 1844; at the Friends' Asylum approximately half of all the inmates attended a series of chemistry lectures in 1841, and three years later a class dealing with unspecified subject matter was inaugurated.

As at other hospitals, the Eastern State Hospital provided Sunday religious services for the patients if they wished to go, with chaplains serving one month each in rotation. In 1855 the chaplain, by then a paid official, was required to be at the asylum one afternoon a week at least and not more than two "to perform such religious services or give such religious instruction as the Superintendent may on the occasion think expedient." Just as he thought religion could prevent insanity, Galt believed it could help cure it. A patient might receive several benefits from attending a sermon: he had to exercise self-control; he gained self-respect at being permitted to hear the clergyman; and his mind was diverted from morbid thoughts. But clergymen had to know how to preach to mental patients; Galt had to caution one "as to sectarianism, as to future punishment & as to long sermons."

In his endorsement of occupational therapy, a cornerstone of moral treatment, Galt more than most psychiatrists stressed the psychological rather than physiological advantages. The insane could benefit from all kinds of work, he believed. The important thing was that their spirits would be lifted and their distrust allayed by the kindness and concern that the provision of work, as well as amusement, evidenced. Further, labor as well as amusement calmed patients and diverted them from morbid thoughts. When asked how many of his patients might be influenced to work if he had "suitable rooms, suitable occupations & suitable industrial supervisors," Galt answered, "I doubt not . . . that our workers would be still further increased in number if we possessed addition in supervision. . . . The number [of supervisors] should only be limited by the funds of an asylum & . . . if each Patient had one of these companions the ratio [of companions to patients] would not be too large."

In his second report Galt maintained that out of 125 inmates all but 20 old and sick ones were engaged in some sort of occupation, a high rate in comparison with successful American mental hospitals, which usually employed no more than about 40 to 50 percent. After 1842 he did not supply statistics on occupational therapy. Galt's apparent success probably can be accounted for by his calling "occupation" any activity, no matter how brief or desultory; this included reading, for example. Much of the actual work involved the male patients' doing "various little offices about the institution," such as helping in the garden, woodyard, and around the premises, cleaning their rooms, and making shoes and instruments of restraint like waistbands and mittens. The women sewed, producing cotton and flannel shirts, bed and pillow ticking, rugs, and other items; they also cleaned their rooms. Later Galt added carpentry, leatherworking, and broommaking. One year, for example, patients made articles to be exhibited at a fair in Richmond, including two bed quilts that were the "admiration of the town" of Williamsburg; as a reward Galt gave the quiltmakers a huge plum cake, for which they came, "much pleased," to his house to thank him.

All this work, Galt insisted, was done primarily as therapy, secondarily for economic benefit to the hospital, an order of priority, he hinted, not always followed before his appointment. With control over his patients' activities now in his hands, he could combine occupation in a "harmonious union" with principles of treatment founded on knowledge of man's fixed and immutable nature. He never used compulsion, he reported, though his private case histories noted that some patients were forced to work—and with good results; in one instance the patient grew "worse from not having shoes to work at."

At other hospitals, including the Western State Hospital, the predominant forms of occupational therapy were farming and gardening, valued for the assumed benefits of physical labor in the open air and the supposed spiritual superiority of the pastoral life as well as for their economic contribution. The directors of the Eastern State Hospital acquired additional land for vegetables and dairy farming and patients were allowed to keep chickens; but such work remained at a minimum and the acreage owned by the hospital continued to be small (twenty acres by 1843, in comparison with sixty-five at the Western State Hospital and little increase thereafter) so that the patients' diet remained low in vegetable products.

During his early years Galt placed more faith in the therapeutic value of mechanical and craft occupations such as shoemaking and sewing than in farming. In his 1843 reorganization plan he suggested, with little result, paying more attention to farming as a financial aid (an idea he soon gave up). Later he proposed, also unsuccessfully, to have a farm for the sick, "the torpid and the labouring." The directors did authorize in 1849 the construction of a greenhouse; finally their intention to buy a tract of land near the asylum useful for farming or grazing purposes was thwarted in 1860 by the veto of the governor, who in this particular case had to give permission.

A possible obstacle to the introduction of extensive agriculture was the townsmen's fear of competition. Some merchants of Williamsburg earned a good deal of money supplying the hospital with its ample provisions, as did its treasurer. Any extension of agriculture at the hospital would reduce their business. Moreover, one should not underestimate the significance of work already being done by patients for staff, directors, and other townsmen, a practice that at the same time alienated people in the community who resented the competition of hospital labor. A staff member accused of employing patients on his land replied that this was the only way of getting them to work, and Galt noted that a director "ran around the street to persuade me not to remove a patient . . . very servicible [*sic*] to him in working, to which I consented." An attempt to limit patients to work only at the asylum unless expressly directed otherwise by the superintendent finally succeeded in 1855. This would be something less than effective, since Galt was not likely to refuse the directors' request for help, and he did not object to having patients work for persons unconnected with the asylum.

[4]

At first Galt ran Eastern State as a largely open hospital, that is, most patients could move about with little restraint. There was no wall around the grounds, nearly all male patients and some females went "unattended and at will about the neighborhood," and officers could take patients on outings in order to give both a respite from hospital routines. Despite the obvious dangers, Galt felt that these policies were good for the patients' mental health and kept them happy; the demented patients improved "from the liberty allowed them. . . . They never pretended to run away." But some caused trouble. One "bothered so many persons in town by talking to them pertinaciously" that Galt had to direct him not to go down town again, and another one knocked at the door of "Mr. W. P." Such an offender "should be forthwith confined" as he would certainly not "be single" in his interruptions.

Allowing patients to go out alone was probably disadvantageous, Galt eventually decided. Not only might townspeople be disturbed, but unless a sane person went along to distract the patients they would brood over old ideas. When, therefore, a Williamsburg judge prohibited patients from making solo excursions out of the hospital on the ground that "no patient was safe without some one attending him," Galt approved, feeling "relieved . . . from the pressure of a load of responsibility." At the same time the decision did not interfere with his "sense of right and of humanity," because he had not been the one to ask the grand jury to take up the issue. Who did ask, and why, he did not say. This ruling of 1851 evidently did not have full effect. Harmless patients still walked into town, and Galt told the hospital's officers that if they let patients go "beyond the premises [they] must . . . be responsible, & the same hold[s] good as to patients employed by persons in town."

Galt also came to endorse the idea of a full wall around the hospital, with a gatekeeper, to regulate patients' movements. In justification he pointed out that having a public street run, as it did, directly through the hospital grounds prevented control of the male patients, some of whom should not be at liberty but did slip into the street and go off on their own. This circumstance led also to the intrusion of the public and the prying curiosity of the idle; and until Galt put a stop to it, numerous dogs invaded the grounds. Finally the directors were able to take possession of the public street and buy a private lot on the premises, so that the entire hospital lands would be under their control. Rules about movement into and out of the grounds remained strict. In 1860 authorization for anyone living in the hospital to leave its enclosure was required from the superintendent or, in his absence, the steward. Only the president of the board, the superintendent, and the mayor of the town had power to give written consent for anyone (except board members and physicians, who did not need it) to be admitted within the gates.

Galt's qualms extended to the practice of allowing patients to go out with staff members, a privilege he did not forbid but disapproved of because he would be blamed for any accidents. Besides, since attendants now took inmates for walks regularly within the hospital grounds, outside excursions were no longer necessary. On the other hand he acknowledged that "even if an accident happened, being granted this privilege [of supervised outings] might hinder the patients from eloping and thus prevent accidents which might ensue from elopments of patients from their dissatisfaction with the close restrictions of the Asylum."

Earlier he had complained that the hospital had so few escapes (one in nine years) because patients had not enough freedom, at the expense of their recovery. What was the point of restricting their liberty in order to prevent escapes if thereby cure was hindered? The price of therapeutic treatment was taking risks, for only so would patients have the opportunity to act like and eventually be transformed into sane people. A policy of wide latitude was therefore essential even if it provoked public criticism. Yet Galt did worry about such criticism and felt concerned enough about the risks to modify his policies if not his beliefs, albeit he felt guilty about the switch.

Galt also changed his mind—this time becoming less restrictive—on a related subject, one that claimed great attention from medical superintendents before the Civil War: restraint versus nonrestraint. Like the rest of his colleagues in the United States, he refused to endorse the principles of the Englishman Robert Gardiner Hill, made popular in England by Dr. John Conolly. Hill and Conolly insisted that mental hospitals abandon all mechanical means of controlling patients, except in very unusual cases. Such a policy, they maintained, would in turn eliminate the need for restraint—strait jackets, mittens, wristbands, and even the more acceptable manual control by attendants—for it would force the staff to pay close attention to the patients, treat them with more kindness, and introduce occupational therapy and a host of other measures that would reduce violent behavior in nearly all cases. Enthusiastic nonrestraint advocates even argued that restraint was never needed in a properly conducted institution.

Galt would not adopt the theory of nonrestraint because he considered it extreme. A physician must never, in principle, surrender the right to employ whatever methods proved useful or necessary, he insisted in 1842. Who knew but that occasionally one might need to apply mechanical control, even in the best hospitals? Happily though, he reported, the simplest and gentlest methods worked best, and nothing such as blows or stripes was permitted at the Eastern State Hospital. There the only means of mechanical restraint ordinarily applied were mittens and wristbands, and those infrequently. Even these rare instances would decline further when a new wing went up and better organization of patients was instituted. Yet, at the same time, Galt replied to the inquiry from the state legislature that he had tried the "ducking stool," or plunge bath, four or five times and found that it tranquilized the patient and was followed by a refreshing sleep; he thought it was perhaps preferable to either the douche or the composing chair (probably Rush's invention, which held a seated patient immobile).

The real issue was Galt's unwillingness to abandon punishment and restraint as significant parts of his system of control. He still thought physical restraint was indicated when patients became violent and that it then served a therapeutic purpose: ". . . very little mental irritation can be at that time produced [by restraints], because the patient hardly notices them; and instead of irritating, by silently preventing the external display of a morbid feeling, they tend to diminish it."

Still, like other American asylum superintendents, he felt the pressure of the English nonrestraint movement, which gained much publicity in the United States. American physicians feared that if they did not reduce greatly or altogether abandon mechanical means of restraint they would face public disapproval, especially in light of the long heritage of cruelty to the mentally ill and the need to overcome mistrust of mental hospitals. They also felt that they had to prove themselves just as capable as their British colleagues of controlling patients without harsh measures.

By March 1844 Galt was noting that only one patient had been under restraint "for some time," and the next year, that some patients were "more easily managed without than with restraints." He described nonrestraint as a great step forward in psychiatry and listed four arguments against restraint: it tended to irritate patients (an about-face from his earlier position); it hindered treating them like sane people; it excited and disturbed those who witnessed it applied to others; and finally, it was the lazy man's out and could thereby easily supplant more humane measures. Solitary confinement, favored by some nonrestraint advocates, was inadvisable because the patient should not be removed from objective influences, such as labor, that helped reduce his excitement. If a patient annoyed others he could be placed in a large room or a court; when in rare cases seclusion was advisable he suggested that the patient be moved frequently from room to room so that he remained no more than a few hours in any one place. In the same report Galt noted that new patients, if violent, would usually be isolated and restraint used if necessary; the previous year the directors had ordered him to have strong rooms fitted up in the west building, facilities not uncommon even in enlightened institutions practicing a modified form of nonrestraint.

In 1853 Galt described the nonrestraint system at the Lincoln Lunatic Asylum in England for his colleagues in the Medical Superintendents' Association. The staff's "patient forebearance . . . and the steady adherence to a sort of moral expectation, instead of endeavoring to cut short the excitement or to repress it by sedative action, deserves at least due attention from every lover of truth," he wrote, even if they unwisely gave up some valuable remedies. The disuse of restraint and the abandonment of seclusion impressed him most. Galt, flexible of mind and always interested in new ideas, presented a much fairer picture of British nonrestraint practices than did other American asylum superintendents, who were generally hostile and defensive on the subject, especially as the British tended toward sharp criticism of psychiatry in the United States.

Though Galt never subscribed fully to nonrestraint as a theory or went as far in his practice of it as did the English, his reports repeatedly maintained that the Eastern State Hospital eschewed mechanical controls. In his article on the Lincoln Asylum he wrote, ". . . by not keeping up too strictly the closing of doors, and other means of classification, we have observed very good effects produced, in warding off the constraining air of confinement," and he exhorted his "lady officers" in 1854 to "try to diminish personal restraint." Stribling, visiting the Eastern State Hospital in 1851, "seemed struck . . . with the small number of patients under restraint, & said he was in favor of it."

Galt would still use confinement and shower baths as punishment or to calm a violent patient; as at many hospitals, a patient's promise to behave usually sufficed to stop this treatment. The records show that excited patients were also secluded in their rooms; there was no mention of moving them about. A suicidal patient who twice jumped into a creek received jalap and a rubdown and was placed in confinement; the promise of good behavior freed another from a "continued course" of baths. Galt ordered a woman patient to be showered if she continued to misbehave. The same fate met one patient who broke his night vessel and threw the contents out the window, and three other patients who "had been excited & complaining for some days." Once Galt foiled an escape by taking away the patient's clothing at night.

Though these measures were not the same as devices applied directly to restrict the patient's movement, such as the strait jacket, the use of physical punishment of any kind violated the spirit of nonrestraint. Yet Galt did recognize the value of a firm, outspoken, but undogmatic commitment to reducing restraint. And he did come, earlier and more fully than any of his better-known contemporaries, to acknowledge the significant contribution made by the British nonrestraint movement to the better care of mental patients.

[5]

The transformation that Galt, working with the directors, was able to effect at the Eastern State Hospital in only a short time was noted by a state Senate committee visiting the hospital in 1845, four years after he took charge. They found it in an "agreeable and unexpected condition . . . a charity now worthy of Virginia and of which she has just reason to be proud." The remodeling, refurbishing, and expansion (including the removal of iron grating from the windows) and the reforms introduced by an intelligent board of directors and an enlightened superintendent had worked "a complete metamorphosis" in the condition of the inmates and in the building, which had been given a "grand, imposing and beautiful appearance."

Specifically, the committee found, the patients' rooms were well lit, well ventilated, and well heated; each of the twelve-foot-square cells had an iron bedstead with a neat, clean bed and bedding, and in many instances a piece of rag carpeting made by the patient lay by the bedside. The entire establishment was neat, clean, and free from odor; there were no instruments of coercion or punishment, nor were any patients chained; and the staff was respectable, intelligent, and kindhearted. The patients had a small library, convenient shops for labor, sufficient wholesome food, warm clothing by day, and comfortable lodgings by night, "with the Word of God to peruse." They attended religious worship on Sundays and had the services of a chaplain; "when sick they [have] the attention of the Superintendent, who is an eminent Physician, and the best of care both by day and by night." Occupation, exercise, and amusements were varied, according to patients' taste and inclination. Punishment was disavowed, and the principle was adopted "that if you wish to benefit the insane you must love him and devote yourself to him." The Eastern State Hospital no longer presented "the gloomy and cheerless aspect of a prison, on the contrary it wears the pleasing and inviting appearance of comfort." The legislature had well spent its money there.

A good deal of Eastern State's relative well-being derived from the continuous expansion of its buildings and the relatively small demands made on it by the mentally ill, who did not flock to it in great numbers. Galt insisted that "a high standard of comfort" proved best in the care and cure of the insane, that patients reacted positively to pleasant surroundings and negatively to unpleasant ones. Although he did make compromises when he could not have his way, in principle he rejected the traditional emphasis on economy that New England superintendents had helped establish as a norm in state mental institutions. Even with a few hard years during the 1850s, the Eastern State Hospital under John Minson Galt II was never subject to the poverty and overcrowding that became common during that decade in many state hospitals.

Besides the addition of porticoes and verandas to improve the appearance of the hospital and give the patients a place to walk and sit, several new brick structures went up by 1850,* increasing the hospital's capacity to 250 patients. Various additions had been made to the hospital from the 1820s. Except for several outbuildings at the rear—the smokehouse, laundry, kitchen, stable, and other outhouses—expansion had been to the east and west of the main building. By the mid-forties wings had been added laterally to connect it to the east and west buildings erected before 1836 (Figure 5). The main asylum structure consisted of the original central building used as officers' residences, two wings, and then, jutting out at right angles from the wings, east and west buildings that formed three sides of a quadrangle with shade trees and flowers in the center. The whole was planned on the model of the Worcester asylum, regarded by the psychiatric profession as holding first place among state hospitals.

The symmetry of the Eastern State Hospital quadrangle was broken by the separate building for convalescents and quiet, pay-

* It is difficult to know exactly how the Eastern State Hospital looked at any one time, with some exceptions, before 1885. All of the original buildings burned and the later ones have been razed. Colonial Williamsburg researchers have assembled many surviving illustrations of the hospital and sketches of its plan made for insurance policies, all of which are helpful in attempting to reconstruct its appearance and development (see Figure 9). While the present study was being prepared for publication, a photograph was discovered that shows the expanded main building from the south before its loss by fire in 1885 (Figure 10). The various annual reports of the hospital during the 1840s and 1850s also contain some information, most of it unfortunately vague, about the buildings.

ing patients, planned about 1848 and completed by 1850. The so-called Doric building or "White House" was a large structure of three stories and a front porch, its façade similar to that of the old center building. A thirty-foot covered walk connected it with the western transverse wing. Graphic evidence indicates that an identical structure was erected opposite to it and connected to the east wing by a walkway (Figure 6), but documentary evidence puts this construction at a later date.

Off by itself to the southwest behind the main complex stood the three-story "Gothic" building for demented, incurable patients and Negro males, planned and finished about the same time as the Doric building. The Gothic building had "at its northern end two towers about ninety feet tall with sleeping rooms in them. At the top of the western tower was a circular platform with seats thereon. Visitors used to be shown to the top of this tower, from which a grand view of the surrounding country, including the James and York rivers, could be obtained." Because of its isolated site the Gothic building could be a departure from the horizontal, classical architecture of the main group of buildings. It reflected Galt's experimentation with a new trend reported from England in the design of poorhouses and asylums. Requiring no attention to symmetry or other classical rules, the "tudor gothic" style was utilitarian and inexpensive and allowed enough variation to provide architectural interest (Figures 7 and 8).

Galt saw the periodic enlargement of the hospital as essential to his therapeutic system. During the early 1840s Eastern State was under-utilized, and Galt and the directors argued in favor of keeping it so, a situation almost unheard of elsewhere. If accommodations could be kept ahead of demand by enlarging the physical plant, they argued, the hospital would be able to treat all patients soon after their attack of illness and not have to turn away any for lack of room. Since most such cases recovered, no large backlog of incurables would develop for many years and the hospital could remain curative.

To what extent was Galt's hope fulfilled? Did he succeed in creating through his various reforms and plans a therapeutic institution? Here much more was involved than his skill as a physician or the worth of his ideas, however well-intentioned and progressive. Many nonmedical and nonpsychiatric conditions and considerations intervened in and interacted with the system he tried to establish. Some of these were carry-overs from previous years, others stemmed from his own personality and inclinations, still others from politics and economics. All were somewhat interrelated and must be investigated to arrive at a more complete picture of the hospital during Galt's twenty-one-year incumbency.

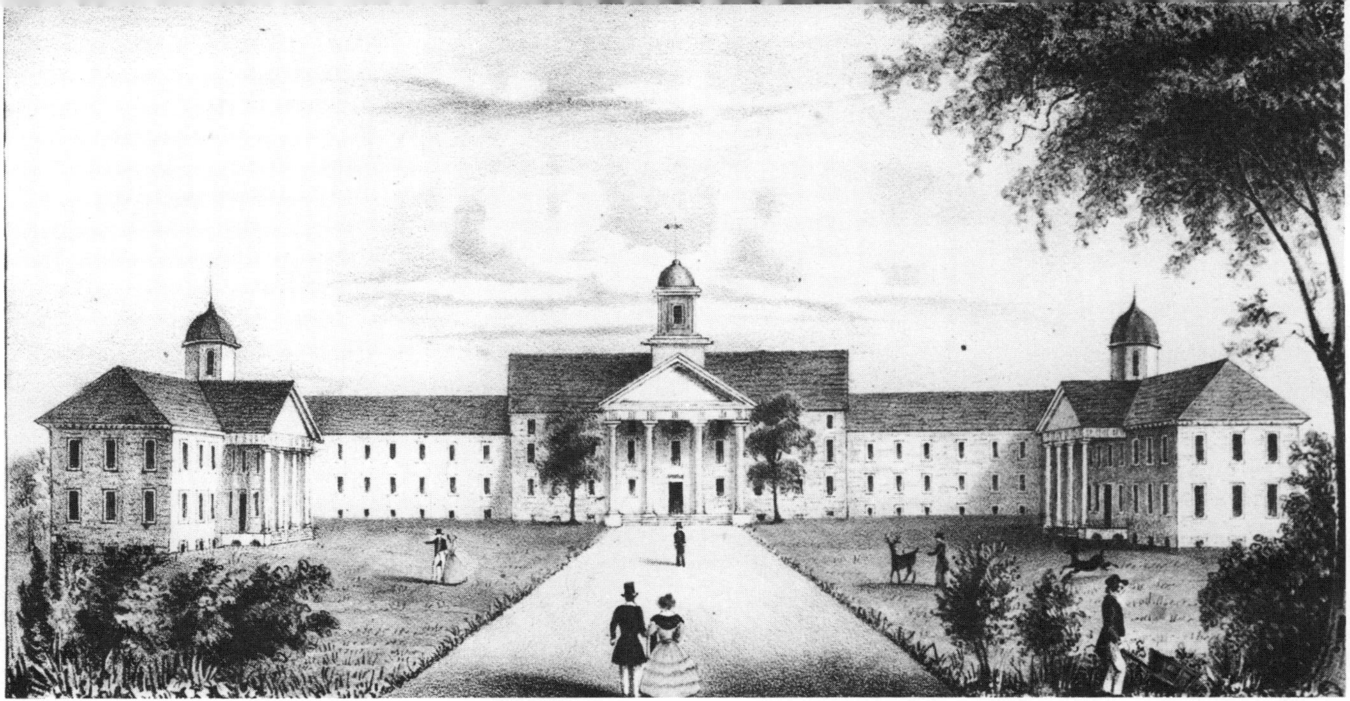

Figure 5
The Public Hospital in the Mid-1840s

A lithograph, several copies of which are in the Galt Family Papers, after an original by Thomas Millington. The approximate location from which this view was made is shown on the site plan, Figure 9.

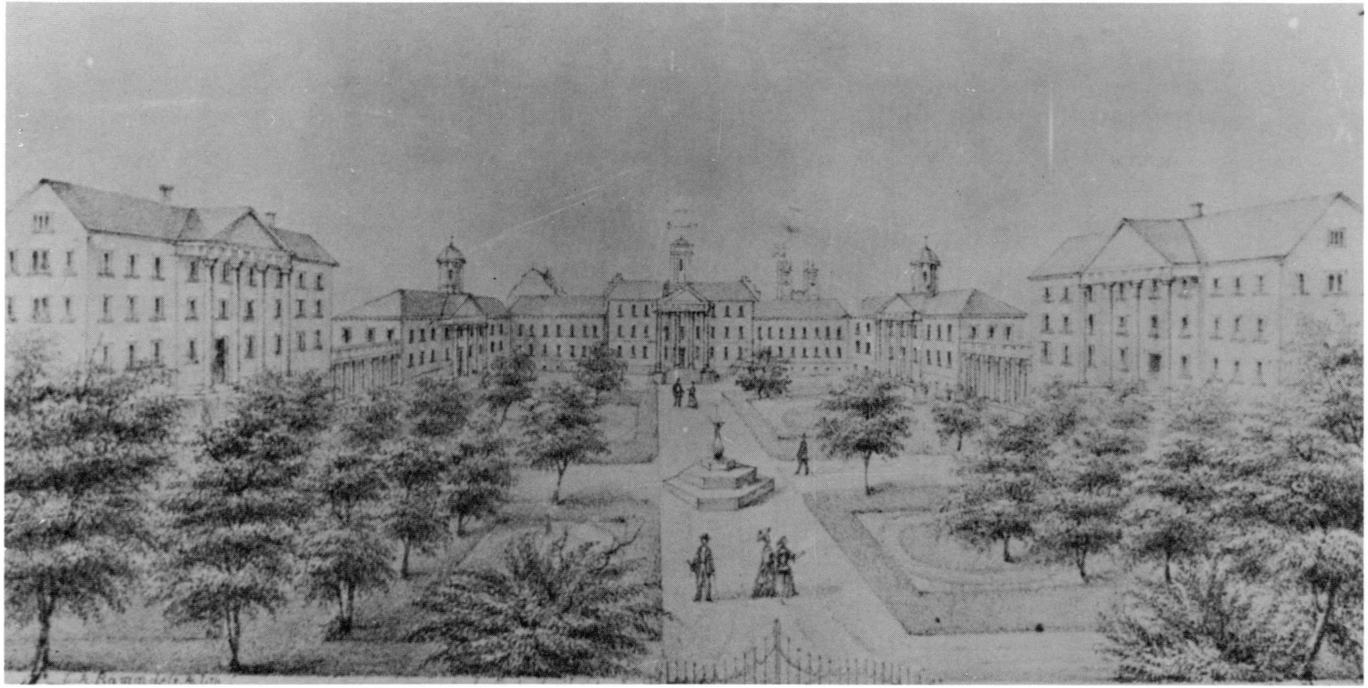

Figure 6

Eastern Lunatic Asylumn, About 1855

When artist and lithographer L. A. Ramn drew this view, he apparently expected the building at the far left to be erected soon and depicted it to match that at the far right. Construction was in fact delayed, no doubt because of the Civil War, until 1869-1872.

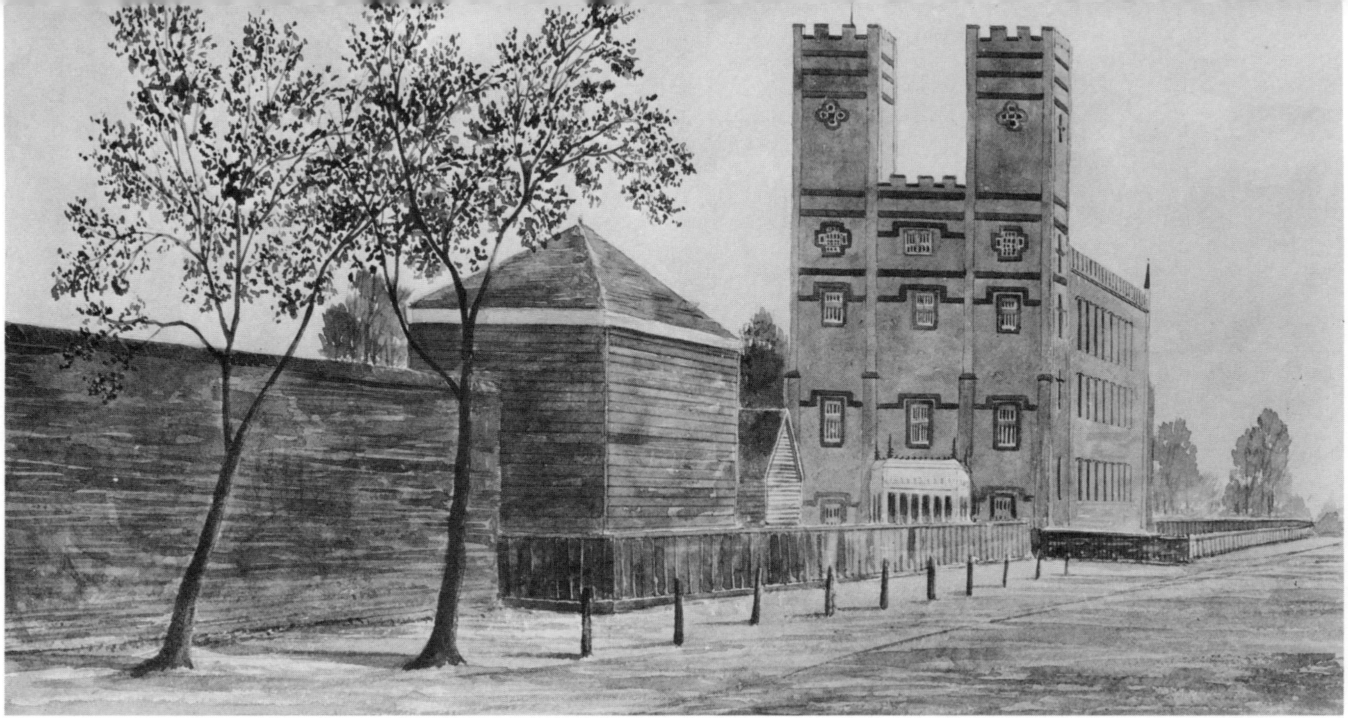

Figure 7
The Gothic Building

A watercolor by Lefevre F. Cranstone, a British artist who painted several Williamsburg scenes about 1860. The building reappears—looking slightly more "Gothic"—in Figure 8.

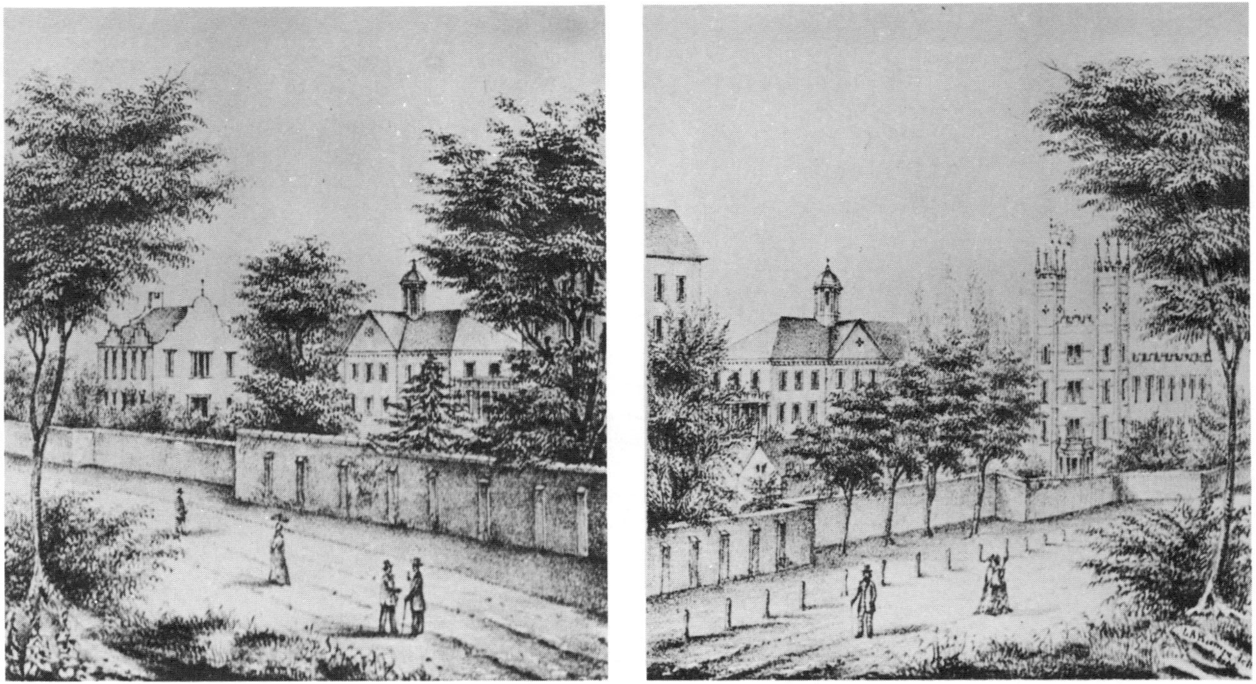

Figure 8

Eastern Lunatic Asylum, About 1855

The view on the *left* shows buildings along the eastern side of the hospital grounds; that on the *right* those on the western side. They are also by L. A. Ramm, and their points of view are shown in Figure 9.

CHAPTER IV

The Struggle for Parity with the Western State Hospital 1841-1862

[1]

AMONG the most important and persistent obstacles to John Minson Galt II's full success in converting the Eastern State Hospital into a superior institution were the composition of its patient population and the closely related problem of competition from the Western State Hospital at Staunton.

Both hospitals had been established on the same basis, open to all classes, rich and poor, white and free black; only slaves seem to have been excluded. Neither was, nor had either ever been, a purely pauper institution. But people came to view the Williamsburg hospital as such, partly because it had always taken free blacks as patients (a policy unique in American mental hospitals, North or South) and as a rule had admitted whites in order of application, regardless of their economic status or length of illness.

The Western State Hospital was from the beginning selective. It not only refused to take Negroes but favored recently ill, curable patients. Thus it did not have much room for longstanding cases, who tended to be poverty-stricken persons coming from long sojourns in jails or almshouses. These rejects would then travel at state expense east to Williamsburg where the hospital usually had vacancies, and the authorities felt obliged to take them.

This was an old story that the new law of 1841 had not ended. In eliminating the boundary line of the Blue Ridge Mountains and requiring patients to apply for admission first to the hospital nearest them, the law, instead of helping the Eastern State Hospital, actually worsened the previous situation. Since by 1841 about three-quarters of the state's population lived closer to Staunton than to Williamsburg, the Eastern State Hospital continued to receive the inevitable overflow from Western State. According to Galt the eastern division held about 360,000 to 400,000 people and the western (which then included what is now West Virginia) from 660,000 to 700,000; nearly 250,000 were taken away from the eastern division by the law of 1841.

Since half in the east were blacks and mostly slaves, this left only about one-third or one-fourth of the state's white population as a source of primary applicants for the Eastern State Hospital. Further, the law came just when the hospital was expanding facilities, so that the area from which it was to take patients contracted while its capacity expanded. Insufficient applications from its own jurisdicion forced Eastern State to admit those rejected by Western State, which, having an excess of applicants, could choose the best prospects and leave the others to Williamsburg.

In 1842, for example, the Eastern State Hospital had only 97 patients when it could hold some 120; the year before, Western State Hospital had to reject about 120 applications; and the United States census of 1840 reported Virginia as having 1,048 white lunatics and idiots, with only a few hundred of them in the mental hospitals. The Eastern State Hospital board spoke of having cleared the insane from the prisons in its territory. Perhaps so; but what of those elsewhere in Virginia? Apparently the sheriffs and jailers had "an interest in Keeping [the insane] in their jails on account of the public allowance and unless coerced by . . . law" would not surrender them, said the Williamsburg representative in the House of Delegates. Before the 1840s Virginia sheriffs were not required to send mental cases in prison to a hospital. Since the sheriffs received more than enough to care for these cases ($247 a year, $100 more than the annual cost per patient at the Eastern and Western

State hospitals), they had a financial incentive to keep patients in jail.

The law of 1837 gave the courts discretionary power to send insane persons charged with crime to a mental hospital. Not until 1843, however, when funds were withheld from sheriffs who did not apply each six months for the admission of insane people in their custody, did sheriffs really begin to empty the prisons of the insane, both criminal and noncriminal. In 1848 the legislature required sheriffs to apply monthly. The almshouses, exempted, continued to shelter the insane. The new regulations affected the Eastern State more than the Western State Hospital because the former had so many vacancies and also because Galt felt obligated to honor such applications for humanitarian reasons. Yet these cases, long-term and incurable, were just the sort he wished to avoid.

Further, Superintendent Stribling of Western State, who could avoid them, was able to attract upper-class whites by introducing moral treatment and offering preferential accommodations for a price. Generally the paying patients at his institution lived apart from nonpaying ones, except when a poor man had a genteel upbringing and was thought to benefit from the company of well-to-do patients. Almost every aspect of moral treatment became more and more a description of how the upper classes were treated. The insane, the common argument at the time went, needed to have conditions at the hospital similar to those at home. The poor, therefore, being unaccustomed to such luxuries as good food, fine clothes, nice furniture, carriage rides, and other amusements, would not appreciate or even benefit from them; the rich had to be provided with them.

This is not to say that nonpaying patients were mistreated or deprived of good care; but since moral therapy involved the total environment, the amenities offered to paying patients—a practice common in general hospitals then and today—were significant aspects of treatment that nonpaying patients lacked. Although the Western State Hospital did not become an exclusive enclave for the upper classes—it admitted somewhat less than a third of its patients from this group—it did develop a dual character. Outside Virginia this difference also existed, but usually between the private, nonprofit corporate institutions and the state hospitals, not within a state hospital or among several in one state.

Even while Galt protested Stribling's selective admissions, he consulted him about special provisions for paying patients and then adopted a plan similar to that followed at the Western State Hospital. Hospitals such as the one he superintended, Galt wrote in his 1843 report, which were "designed directly for the insane poor [did] not perhaps require so great a variety of amusements as those intended for the rich: for it [was] always requisite in asylums, to pay regard to the previous habits of patients."

In November of that year the Eastern State Hospital directors had endorsed various policies to this effect. They authorized the purchase of new furniture, including iron bedsteads recommended by Dr. Amariah Brigham, the editor of the *American Journal of Insanity* and superintendent of the Utica State Hospital of New York. The order for a new supply of books, maps, and musical instruments, and Galt's concern about the appearance of the hospital buildings, while fitting his concept of proper therapy, seemed also to be designed to attract paying patients. And now that the hospital would offer more substantial facilities for such persons, the directors could forbid staff members to take paying patients home for private care, though it seems the practice did not stop.

In 1850 "a splendid new building [was] finished for the best class of patients which [was] thought by many to be handsomer than the Gothic building." (This probably referred to the Doric building.) Two grades of paying patients were established in 1843: those in the first paid $15 a month and were the same sort of patients as had previously paid for their keep; those in the second, a new category designed for patients who wanted "a superior order of accommodation," paid a monthly charge of $17. All extra services and accommodations would be paid for according to private agreement between the superintendent and the friends of the patient. The monthly fees were high for a state hospital, where it was customary for paying patients, usually of the lower middle class, to defray their costs, plus a little more. Eastern State Hospital patients paying the higher amount had no exact counterpart in most northern state hospitals. In the North such persons would go to private asylums, of which Virginia had none.

The Eastern State Hospital continued to admit not only white paupers but free blacks, who also could not afford to pay; later, insane slaves were taken and facilities for black patients expanded. These policies helped lower the hospital's status in a class- and race-conscious society. Indeed, Galt's liberalism was sharply criticized by the prominent, long-time head of the psychiatric department of the Pennsylvania Hospital, Thomas Kirkbride, whose opinion was shared by most other superintendents: "The idea of mixing up all colors and all classes, as is seen in one or two institutions of the United States, is not what is wanted in our hospitals for the insane, although it may be regarded by [Galt] as a desirable kind of liberty."

Galt's statement that the directors had made "no difference in their exertions for [blacks] & for the white Population" applied more to admissions than to their condition within the hospital. Nearly all the free blacks sent to the hospital were admitted, but even less than the paupers did they receive the full benefits of moral treatment. When introducing reforms or experimental procedures, Galt generally gave the white males preference; then followed white females, and last, the blacks. However, "no particular strictness" was observed, he said, "in isolating the white from the colored patients; nor . . . [was] there the slightest difficulty . . . originating" from this policy.

He used, though, an old outbuilding once devoted to convalescents for the colored females, who were "thus never in contact ncessarily with the white patients," which was "in all respects the best arrangement for these persons." The black males, half the number of black women, though not segregated from the other patients, were seldom in the wards during the day and therefore had little to do with white patients. In any case, he said, the whites looked upon the black patients much as they did slave servants, particularly as the black patients did much of the work of maintaining their own quarters.

[2]

By the 1840s the Eastern State Hospital came under pressure

from slaveholders to take slaves as patients. Such requests Galt found hard to resist, especially since he believed there were too few mentally ill blacks, slave or free, to warrant establishing a separate asylum. Western State Hospital would not admit even free blacks, on the ground that an integrated asylum would harm both black and white patients, for the whites' normal antipathy to blacks probably increased under the impact of insanity. They should rather be segregated in distinct institutions, Stribling said, or if they had to be in one asylum, in separate buildings.

In 1841 the House of Delegates tabled a motion that the Committee on Lunatic Asylums inquire into the expediency of caring for insane slaves. Five years later Galt and his board obtained a legislative change that permitted them to admit slaves, on condition that no white patients should thereby be excluded from treatment. Galt tried to counter opposition by proposing a separate division or wing for black patients. No harm would come to the whites if their contact with blacks was slight, as Superintendent Woodward had found at Worcester State Hospital. Galt maintained he did not have facilities to take many male slaves but could probably accommodate all the women who needed care.

Slaves would be accepted at the Eastern State Hospital at $1.50 a week, exclusive of clothes and transportation, and placed with free Negro patients. A resolution of the General Assembly on January 11, 1848, required the mental hospitals of Virginia to report on the propriety and costs of making provision for the Negro insane either within or outside their establishments. In replying Galt considered how to insure that no danger or disadvantage to whites would occur; the directors decided that $8,000 would do for the necessary facilities, an amount less than retention of insane blacks in jails would cost. Of two new buildings authorized, one, the Gothic, would have a section for black men. An additional building for black females was requested, to replace their "somewhat ruinous" accommodations.

Eventually more "suitable provision for . . . colored male patients" was required. Placing them in the basement of the Gothic building, with a separate attached yard, Galt wrote in 1857, assured "sufficient isolation if enforced . . . however . . . the white Patients exhibited the strongest inclination to come into the ward where the colored insane were placed, and we therefore determined to ultimately erect an entirely distinct building." But not much harm resulted from such contacts, "if for no other reason, at least from the inconsiderable number [of Negroes] present." The proportion of free black patients fluctuated at about 10 percent from the time the hospital opened and remained so after 1845, and the number of slave admissions could not have been high. In 1862 there were forty black patients out of a total of three hundred, or 13 percent. Increased numbers of blacks, then, could not account for Galt's proposal to segregate the black males fully for the first time.

What probably happened was that the matter became one of legislative and public concern, and he felt obliged to bow to those who feared the mixing of black and white patients. Because the legislature required the hospital to expel insane slaves if there were whites needing treatment, Eastern State discharged some slave patients and as of October 1, 1856, refused to take any more of them. This left rooms in the Negro section empty. Galt, not deeming it "requisite to leave rooms untenanted, when the white insane were languishing in jails," assigned some of the cells to the latter. But he was afraid this action would bring legislative criticism of the hospital. The assembly, he wrote,

> first passes a resolution, very philanthropic to be sure, as though they would provide for the colored insane, whilst still insisting on sending the slaves home, notwithstanding the slight expense involved in their accommodations; and moreover themselves bring on a measure [the mixing of blacks and whites] for which we are prepared for them to censure us.

Galt made exceptions to the law at times. In 1860 he wrote to the president of the Court of Directors, Robert Saunders, about one case. Previously he had, regardless of the availability of white applicants, retained as a patient the slave of a board member and also had taken another slave who had only recently fallen ill and was therefore curable. He wanted now to admit a probably incurable slave of a local widow. To do so would for a long time exclude a white patient, but not to accept the slave would condemn him to remain in jail, a source of great uneasiness to his owner. What should he do? Saunders told Galt to admit him and not to worry about the future. The law might be stretched a bit to give preference to slaves from the immediate neighborhood, especially in cases of great hardship. They must always remember that an asylum was a nuisance in a small town and that every convenience should therefore be offered to its residents.

Galt sympathized with the blacks as suffering human beings and also with the plight of their masters, but any notions of equality or emancipation were anathema to him. Staunch defender of slavery and states' rights, he shared the paternalistic attitudes of well-born Virginians toward the Negro people, who, he believed, could "only be equal to the white by their great cheerfulness & devotion. As the eagle to the sparrow." The small proportion of insane slaves in Virginia as shown by the census of 1840 was "perhaps owing not only to the less degree of mental cultivation, but much also to the absence of all cares for the future, the great depressing influence with the whites." Abolitionists should be warned by the census report that one of every fourteen Negro freedmen in Maine was insane; if the abolitionists attained their goal the Negro would, through misuse of his freedom, suffer a fantastic amount of mental illness. Galt ignored the work of statistician-psychiatrist Edward Jarvis which proved the census figures on insanity to be highly inaccurate.

Galt's insensitivity to the problems faced by slaves and his claim that they did not fear for the future were typical, even in an educated and otherwise sensitive man, of a citizen of a state that in he second quarter of the nineteenth century sold excess slaves into the Deep South cotton country. That he never considered the separation of families and friends, which such commerce inevitably entailed, as conducive to insecurity and anxieties at least among some slaves was a blindness shared by many asylum superintendents, not to speak of laymen, and testifies to the power of racism in both North and South. They saw problems in the Negro's life as arising only from his freedom, not his enslavement. Free blacks suffered more frequently from insanity than slaves, "most probably [because of] their degradation and misery and great tendency to vicious and dissipated habits," Galt wrote.

The theories about insanity among Negroes that were current in the psychiatric profession resembled those concerning lower-class people in general. During the eighteenth century many physicians had assumed that the poor were too busy trying to stay alive and too coarse to suffer from the mental problems that brought on insanity. Such illness allegedly affected primarily the sensitive, civilized, upper classes. Only later, in the mid-nineteenth century, when lower-class patients began to flood the newly established public mental hospitals, did physicians change their minds and consider insanity a special disorder of the so-called vicious, vulgar poor.

In the North the immigrant, non-Protestant poor took the brunt of condemnation. In the South, without the great tides of immigration, the city poor were thought to be particularly subject to insanity, but because of the small numbers of such persons entering the two Virginia hospitals, this subject never received much attention from either Galt or Stribling. Galt did describe the pauper patients sent from Richmond and the large towns of eastern Virginia as in general the worst class of patients, difficult to manage and cure. Their condition was exacerbated, he thought, by the tendency first to seek relief from various local physicians and thus to delay their coming to the Eastern State Hospital until they became incurable.

[3]

In northern state hospitals pessimism about curing the insane began to set in during the 1850s for a variety of reasons. Among the most important were class and religious prejudices, crowded conditions, and insufficient appropriations, all of which made almost impossible the continuance of effective practices. The middle-class Protestant asylum superintendents, disillusioned, frustrated, and ineffective in obtaining more funds, tended to blame the patients themselves for their failure to recover, the urban poor and the allegedly unassimilable immigrants being particularly culpable on account of their poverty, immorality, and heredity.

To the extent that moral treatment survived, it did so primarily in the corporate asylums that could choose their patients and avoid overcrowding. Moral treatment, then, starting out as applicable in theory to all classes of persons, ended as an exclusive prerogative of middle- and upper-class native Americans who could best pay for it and were deemed best able to benefit from it. These attitudes were not confined to American mental hospitals. The historian of Bethlehem Hospital in England writes of its first medical superintendent, appointed in 1853: "Now Dr. Hood had realized from the first that, if he was to attract and retain a more educated and refined class, he must be prepared to offer them something akin to what they were familiar with in their own homes." He thus needed to reduce and even eliminate the poor and criminal element from the hospital.

The situation at the Eastern State Hospital was somewhat different. Though Galt showed evidence of sharing some of the views of his northern colleagues, it would seem that in his case they derived more from a middle-class orientation than from experience at his hospital. He never had the problem of overcrowding, and the hospital usually had enough money to maintain minimum comfort for its inmates and offer them a reasonably pleasant existence. Virginia was still predominantly rural and, compared with states like Massachusetts and New York, sparsely populated. It did not attract the masses of immigrants that deluged the northern coastal cities. Its own oppressed and impoverished class, the blacks, while numerous enough, scarcely posed such an overwhelming problem to its mental hospitals as did the immigrants in the North.

Except for the reception of a few slaves toward the end, the social composition of the patient population at the Eastern State Hospital changed little in the nineteenth century: white patients and staff tended to be ethnically homogeneous, that is, Anglo-Saxon Protestant. Galt and the directors saw the serious problems that the Eastern State Hospital had in regard to curability of patients and to its reputation as related to the socio-economic status of the patients, but the latter were not regarded as inherently incurable because of their status or, in the case of blacks, their color. Blame went instead to their not being sent early enough to the hospital, a condition aggravated by the Western State Hospital's selective admission policies and the failure of local authorities promptly to clear the jails and almshouses of the insane.

Stribling, focusing on more recent cases and on middle- and upper-class patients who would tend to find their way to the hospital faster than the poor, left for the Eastern State Hospital long-standing cases that allegedly would undermine that institution as a therapeutic agency. In protesting against this, Galt retained his optimism that recently ill patients, regardless of social origin, could be cured; he did not seem to lose faith in moral treatment, if only he could have better candidates for it. Yet this system, founded so much on high expectation of cures, could not help being weakened by the nature of the patients. Galt had fairly quickly brought his hospital to the point where treatment given patients differed only slightly from that at Staunton. What counted, though, were results in terms of recoveries.

Galt initially reported greatly increased success in restoring patients. During the first two full years of his administration approximately 53 percent of newly admitted patients were listed as cured. In his first full report (for 1842) he noted that twelve out of thirteen recent cases had recovered within a year (only the premature death of one patient prevented a perfect score): ". . . from such facts . . . I am led to believe that there is no insane institution, either on the continent of Europe, in Great Britain, or in America, in which such success is met with as in our own." Such boasting and exaggerated interpretation of statistics were common among American medical superintendents during the 1840s. But Galt soon had to subdue his pride and finally swallow it. For in the next two years his recovery rates declined to 28 percent of yearly admissions, and though subsequent figures sometimes went above this they never reached the early peak.

Galt admitted that the Eastern State Hospital fell behind the more successful institutions, and he became progressively more shy about publishing the number of cures, preferring to mention only discharges, which included cases sent home for reasons other than their being cured. The available evidence, inconsistent and sparse as it is, indicate that throughout his tenure the hospital restored an average of from 30 to 32 percent of yearly admissions in comparison with something over 40 percent at Western State. By the 1850s the Eastern State Hospital had the reputation among asylum superintendents of being filled with the chronic and demented.

Galt and his board blamed their relatively unsatisfactory record on Stribling's admissions policies and the unfair provision in the 1841 law, which, they complained, was calculated to make their institution a "receptacle of worn out cases." Galt illustrated the effect on his recovery rates by showing that from March 6, 1841, to March 6, 1847, more than 50 percent of those patients coming to Williamsburg without having first sought entry into the Staunton hospital recovered, as compared with less than 20 percent of those initially turned down by the Western State Hospital.

The Eastern State Hospital did not accept the situation passively. Galt and the board fought for years to remedy the injustice they saw in the law and Stribling's interpretation of it. Galt considered this the most important subject that had ever come before the board. If a corrective law did not pass, the hospital would "finally become a mere subsidiary to the western institution." No other public hospital in the United States or Europe, he wrote, experienced the prejudicial territorial division inflicted on Eastern State.

At the end of 1843 Galt began a campaign for new legislation with a petition to the General Assembly asking that the state be divided into two parts by the Blue Ridge Mountains (much as it was before 1841). The Eastern State Hospital would then have enough applicants so that it would not be forced to admit Staunton's rejects. A year later the directors of the Williamsburg hospital appointed a committee of two to go to Richmond "to attend to the interests of the asylum before the committee on lunatic asylums of the General Assembly." Galt was active preparing memoranda, furnishing facts, and corresponding with Stribling, a task he did not relish.

Stribling had news of events in Richmond from friendly state legislators who asked his advice in formulating strategy. The Williamsburg people, in pushing for a new law, one of his friends wrote, alleged that Stribling kept cells in reserve for paying patients and recent cases and could thereby show a higher rate of cures and at a "seeming less cost to the commonwealth." But their scheme would not succeed, for the East would "not commit such a suicidal act as to deprive themselves of the benefit of such an Institution [the Western State Hospital] to gratify the caprice of the folks at Williamsburg." Another member of the House of Delegates informed Stribling that the struggle would be bitter, for eastern delegates had a majority and the Williamsburg men were determined to "make a desperate effort." The westerners succeeded in delaying action, and "Bowden of Wsburg after his failure got out of temper & stormed & swore . . . that they never would cease making application until they got justice." He declared they would "never accept . . . chronic [patients] from west of the Blue Ridge."

Stribling, though maintaining that the Eastern State Hospital petition contained "errors," which he did not specify, evaded a direct response to its charges. He did not wish to become a "party in the matter," and anyway, when his new facilities were completed he would be able to admit all applicants, so that the problem would disappear and with it the need for any change in the law.

From the beginning some legislators, unhappy about the controversy, wanted to see it settled informally. Galt agreed to meet Stribling, who replied that he had always wanted amicable relations with the Eastern State Hospital and that the true interests of both institutions coincided. He then rejected any new division of territory as unacceptable to both, but he would "acquiesce in a repeal of this section [of the 1841 law] thereby leaving it discretionary with officers & individuals, to convey insane citizens, from whatever portion of the state, to that asylum which they may prefer." Such a policy would place the two hospitals on the same footing and give the taxpayers the right to choose between them. Stribling's chief legislative informant, John G. Fulton, favored this proposal because the Eastern State Hospital men had made a convincing case and there was "Great Complaint." Nothing came of the compromise offer, however.

Stribling finally answered Galt's charges in a letter to the Virginia legislature dated January 6, 1845. (His first letter on the subject in 1843 was lost before many lawmakers could see it, but he apparently felt no need to replace it until 1845.) A mental hospital should not be judged, he said, on the absolute number of patients restored but rather on the ratio of cured to recent cases, so that in this regard the Eastern State Hospital could do as well as any other institution even if it received few curable cases. As for the financial burden of sending patients from the west to Williamsburg, the cost was compensated for by those who now could come to Staunton instead of traveling a great distance to the Eastern State Hospital. He denied admitting only recent cases and asserted that where equal chances of recovery existed the rich were discriminated against in favor of poor patients, not the reverse. Moreover, during the period from March 6, 1841, to December 31, 1843, under the 1841 law only eighteen cases went from west of the Blue Ridge to the Williamsburg hospital, and the Western State Hospital accepted all applicants.

Stribling's arguments are not altogether convincing. If the Eastern State Hospital received only a few curable cases out of new admissions, certainly the public could be excused if it considered the recovery of even a high proportion of these patients a sign of failure, especially when Stribling boasted in his annual reports of curing more than 40 percent of *all* admissions. The directors and superintendent of the Williamsburg hospital could hardly be expected to be satisfied with a "success" that would ultimately fill the institution with incurables. Further, as many of the recently ill indigent patients would first go to jails or almshouses while those of the upper classes could go directly to hospitals, Western State faced few occasions to choose between the two groups. Well-to-do-patients, besides, paid their own way and lived in special quarters set aside for them, hence reducing the accommodations available for non-paying patients.

Galt answered Stribling's arguments in several memoranda that spoke of the difficulties of dealing with the paupers and incurables who crowded into the Eastern State Hospital as a result of Stribling's discretionary policy. He also noted the rise in the death rate of his establishment occasioned by the forced reception of aged patients, a point difficult to verify because mortality figures fluctuated greatly as a consequence of epidemics. During the hospital's early years the annual death rate tended to drop. In the period

1798–1810 it was probably 18 percent, from 1811 through 1823, approximately 12 percent (remaining at about that level until A. D. Galt's death in 1841). During the years 1843–1852 an average of 7.59 percent died, the lowest figure being 3.82 in 1847 and the highest 11.62 in 1849. In 1843, when Galt wrote, it had reached 10.37, as compared with 4.91 percent at the Western State Hospital, where the average annual rate from 1828 to 1841 was 5 percent, an acceptable average in well-run hospitals. The whole situation tended to influence curable and easily managed patients to choose the Staunton hospital to avoid being incarcerated with hopeless old people at Williamsburg. It was consequently, hard for the Eastern State Hospital to build good will even within its own territory, let alone outside it.

Despite serious reservations, Galt at first supported a measure proposed by Stribling to the state legislature that would sanction preference in admissions to curable patients and allow the hospitals to send home old, harmless incurables. In 1845 Galt switched his position, arguing that incurable patients did poorly when sent home; he also doubted the propriety of such a policy. That he perhaps overstated the effect of Stribling's admissions policies on the Eastern State Hospital is indicated by his private comment that "the size of Virginia & the natural putting-off mind of Virginians, leads to few recent cases being brought to the Hospitals for the insane."

Stribling did not respond to Galt's suggestion for a united call upon the General Assembly to return to a firm division of territory. Galt, assisted by his directors and the Williamsburg representatives in the assembly, still met with no success. Year after year he discussed the issue in his annual reports and sent, through the Court of Directors, petitions and messages to the assembly and even went there to argue in person, all to no effect. He eventually conceded to the directors that they should ask for a much smaller territory for the Williamsburg hospital, and to Stribling he proposed that their respective institutions be granted territory proportionate to their capacity to receive white patients: 220 for Staunton and 150 for Williamsburg.

Finally, Galt sought a law prohibiting a hospital from discriminating among applicants unless both institutions were crowded. "I understood [Stribling] to acquiesce in such an arrangement," Galt reported. "I do not know however, whether the friends of the Western Asylum will approve the change." He wanted a legislative decision on whether the hospital he superintended did or did not have the right to select patients. He may have hoped the assembly would deny this power to him and thereby also indirectly to the Staunton institution.

The only apparent accomplishment of all these efforts was to put the Western State Hospital on the defensive about its admission policies and to gain for Galt legislative permission, also extended to Stribling, to admit paying patients from other states at four dollars a week, exclusive of clothes and transportation. This would enable Galt to make use of his excess facilities, raise the status of the hospital, and provide a place in the South to send southerners from states without mental hospitals. Circulars were distributed soliciting patients and describing the Eastern State Hospital, including laudatory endorsements from President John Tyler (a Williamsburg man), the Protestant Episcopal bishop of Virginia, the president of the College of William and Mary, and Dr. Amariah Brigham.

[4]

The controversy between the two state mental hospitals of Virginia continued into the 1850s. In 1854 the Eastern State directors complained to the legislature that the influx of Western State rejects was causing their institution economic hardship, draining its transportation fund, and straining its operating budget, especially since prices of goods and slave labor were so high. They requested that a third asylum be established west of the Allegheny Mountains to ease the financial pressure on the Williamsburg hospital. The board then refused to take rejects from Staunton unless given evidence that Stribling had no room for them; they also wanted information about the condition of such persons, who were so often difficult to cure and care for.

Stribling would not give this information, insisting that his word on vacancies should suffice. The Eastern State Hospital president, Lemuel J. Bowden, who had campaigned for a change in the law in the House of Delegates during the 1840s, led the fight, declaring that Galt should reject out of hand Stribling's leftovers. But the Court of Directors feared the law would not support that position, and Galt explained that because four-fifths of all applications to mental hospitals in Virginia were addressed first to Staunton, the Eastern State Hospital could not refuse old cases when it had unused facilities. Finally the frustrated directors ordered that preference of admission be given patients from the "Eastern District & favorable cases." In his report for 1854 Galt commented bitterly on the "miserable, contracted policy which has characterized the enactments regulating the admission of patients in this State."

The year before, Galt began to push for a new plan that would, though he did not say so, solve the problem. It was based on the desirability of separating the sexes in different hospitals, an idea then held by several other psychiatrists. The state of Virginia would establish a third asylum in the far west that would take patients of both sexes from beyond the Alleghenies. Then all female patients living to the east would go to Staunton and all males to Williamsburg, a change that would permit the latter to increase its population twofold. The Eastern State Hospital board incorporated Galt's proposal in its suggestion to the General Assembly in 1854 for a third asylum.

A new institution was built at Weston (later part of West Virginia) and opened in 1859, but Galt's scheme for dividing the sexes was never adopted. The Western State Hospital continued to be selective, to the point where the governor intervened to inform Stribling of repeated complaints about it. In 1857 the much higher annual income received from paying patients at the Staunton hospital ($17,000–$18,000) than at the Williamsburg hospital ($2,500) testified, as the General Assembly was told, to the comparatively large pauper population in the latter institution.

Why, despite the obvious injustices perpetuated by the 1841 act, did Galt and his board fail in their attempt to have the legislature redistrict the territories from which the two hospitals drew patients? A large part of the answer was the proficiency of Stribling and his board in gaining legislative and public support. From the first, Stribling educated the governor about the great success of his institution, and he and his board did all the right things to win the favor of state legislators. They befriended them; did them services; sent them their annual reports (which they began to publish several years earlier than did the Eastern State Hospital); and welcomed them to visit the hospital, where they would hear about its high rates of recovery.

A well-wishing friend whose slaves were employed at the Eastern State Hospital suggested that Galt emulate Stribling. "When we parted in Petersburg I promised to write . . . & give you the names of several gentlemen who had desired me to procure for them the *report of the Lunatic Asylum*," he wrote. Then followed the names of members of the House of Delegates, including Mr. M., a "delegate-elect," "a good but rather silly fellow," to whom Stribling had, as was his custom, sent the Western State Hospital report, and who might "think hard of it" unless he received one from Galt. The Western State men made "every effort to conciliate & gain popularity with Members of the Legislature." Stribling's activities did not go unremarked by the Eastern State Hospital's directors. It was observed privately to Galt that Stribling "had more cunning" than he did.

Stribling's success led to further success, especially as he had the advantage of age and experience, being nine years older than the youthful Galt and five years longer in his superintendency. Legislators would send their insane friends and relatives to Staunton, not Williamsburg, and they came to know and respect Stribling as a physician and friend. It was not stated openly, but some of them thought that the Eastern State Hospital wanted changes in the law because of its inability to compete with the Staunton hospital in patient care rather than inequitable admissions policies and a favorable geographical situation.

A perhaps typical opinion was expressed in a letter to the clerk of the Western State Hospital in 1841: "I am . . . advised that the institution at Staunton is much more favorable for the cure of such unfortunate [insane] persons than [is] Williamsburg." More revealing is a letter Stribling received in 1860 from a newly appointed director of the Eastern State Hospital, W. R. Garrett. Claiming to be ignorant about mental hospitals he asked Stribling, known "throughout our Union for . . . skill in the management of that unfortunate class of persons," to answer some questions about medical administration that would come up at the next directors' meeting. Stribling refused to undercut Galt and suggested that Garrett take his own superintendent's opinion as authoritative. (At least he did so in the first half of his answer; the second is torn off.)

Stribling's reputation did have a solid basis. Not as thoughtful or scholarly as Galt in theoretical matters, he was a capable administrator and devoted physician presiding over a well-run hospital and able to gain his patients' love and respect. He kept in close contact with former inmates, asking them about their condition and replying to their letters. One set of letters speaks of a patient who had been in both Virginia mental hospitals; the correspondent observes that Galt wrote frequently but not so much or in such detail as Stribling. Not that Galt was any the less regarded by his patients. The point is that Stribling's success involved more than an ability to ingratiate himself with politicans and the public.

The disagreement over admission policies did not prevent the two men from cooperating occasionally on mutually agreeable projects, especially at the beginning of their acquaintance,* and in the late 1850s some degree of rapprochement between them occurred. Stribling visited the Eastern State Hospital, and he and Galt went to a party together. Despite these and other contacts they never developed warm relations; Stribling seems to have considered Galt a queer duck while Galt continued to feel aggrieved.

---

* In the history of American psychiatry Stribling is probably best known as the initiator, with Samuel B. Woodward, of the Association of Medical Superintendents of American Institutions for the Insane. Stribling corresponded with Galt about founding the Association in 1844 and eventually both men joined eleven other physicians to do so. They also worked together in an exchange of annual reports with European asylum superintendents. With the approval of Woodward, James Barnard, a Boston merchant, suggested that American superintendents give him their reports to be exchanged for similar ones from Europe; the European reports would be circulated among superintendents in the United States and all interested parties would thus have access to news of latest developments abroad. In Barnard's letter there is mention of a fifteen months' trip through Europe when he apparently learned about an association of British physicians associated with mental hospitals, so that it is possible that Woodward first got the idea of forming an American association from Barnard.

[5]

The superiority of the Western State Hospital included its physical plant as well, considered so important in creating a healing environment and appealing to the proper kind of patients. Through continual expansion the Eastern State Hospital had enough room for patients, and during the 1840s Galt had managed to acquire some new furnishings and to make the entire establishment more attractive. As in all other matters, he had kept up with the latest writings and developments in hospital architecture and tried to turn them to practical advantage. Yet despite his knowledge of the "best standard" of his day and his concern for a comfortable and visually pleasing institution, he made adjustments for reasons of economy, and his new buildings lacked some facilities considered essential in many state hospitals. The ideal institution, he believed, had only one story, but this was too expensive and so he had to settle for three, not two, as Kirkbride, the building expert, recommended. For good lighting only one side of a hallway should be used for patients' rooms; Galt accepted having rooms on both sides. Hot water heating cost too much, so fireplaces and stoves had to do.

He found good arguments to support his compromises. Since most of the existing buildings had two stories, an exception or two could do no harm and would provide additional space. The short distance the hallways ran insured light to them. In some of his new buildings he supplied more light and air by having the upstairs hallway or "gallery" end in a large room that would serve as a "pleasant sitting and workroom" for the women; on the lower story three central arches replaced what otherwise would have been given over to patients' rooms. Convalescents enjoyed the sofa, ottomans, piano, mirrors, and other comforts in this arched apartment. Later Galt maintained that the patients got plenty of light and air from spending much of their time outdoors. In any case, gas lighting was introduced at the end of 1855.

Generally Galt followed the practice of allotting one room to each patient, but in 1845, influenced by the report of another asylum, he proposed adding twenty-seven more pauper patients by placing forty males in wards with several beds each and without any night attendants; similar changes in the women's wards would raise the number of patients to about two hundred, all without appreciable increase in capital expenditure. Perhaps more sober consideration convinced him that this plan was shortsighted, since he never implemented it. In his last buildings he had a few "associate dormitories," rooms where two to four or sometimes more persons slept. These were primarly suicidal patients who would tend not to harm themselves if other persons were present, a measure suggested by the French psychiatric authority J. E. D. Esquirol. Dormitories also served well for "melancholy, timid patients, who are afraid of being left alone at night" as well as those tending to destroy their clothes and other objects.

As for the heating system, hot water might be the best method, Galt admitted, but the cost was prohibitive and in the warm climate of Williamsburg it was really not necessary. Experience during the cold winters of 1855/56 and 1856/57 confirmed his opinion that open fireplaces sufficed for the great majority of patients. Only a few who threw off their blankets at night should have other forms of heat; for them he suggested one ward for men and one for women warmed by hot water or steam.

In this way, too, the few inmates inclined to burn their clothes or sit too near the fire would also be protected. This concession must have come from unhappy experience; at one time, for example, he discovered a patient to be frostbitten who should have been "placed during the cold weather in one . . . of the upper rooms: the females have never been . . . affected, from the care taken in wrapping and tying blankets about their extremities." Over a year later this same patient "died suddenly, with disease of lungs; probably apoplexy of lungs."

The new buildings constructed for the Williamsburg hospital during Galt's administration were by comparison with many northern institutions and even with its rival at Staunton apparently below standard, but Galt and the directors never dared ask for the considerable sums required to construct them adequately. By the late 1850s they were petitioning the legislature for money to repair "the ruinous condition of the buildings" owing to a defective drain and sewer system. A friend told Galt in 1860 that the "slightest comparison of the [Eastern State Hospital] with the Asylum at Staunton will show the *necessity* and the *right* which [Eastern State Hospital] has to claim aid and improvement from the state." Unfortunately he knew of no legislator making a special effort to win support for the needed changes.

Certain of them seemed essential: a better supply of water and drainage of the "slop & waste water thrown above ground"; change in the place to deposit sweepings, ashes, and other waste then thrown south of the woodyard wall and producing "very bad odours in evaporation"; better grading of the front yard or lawn; provision of furnaces in the basement room instead of the coal grate used for heating; and finally, "in ventilation also a good deal might be done to advantage." Conditions deteriorated during the Civil War; afterward the first civilian superintendent made similar criticisms and spoke of female patients who, because of an unusable furnace, must sleep all night in cold rooms.

In asking for funds for construction, Galt and the directors did not cite amounts, which they felt certain the General Assembly would reject as extravagant no matter how essential to the proper care of the insane. They tended to be less conservative in their requests, normally presented in annual reports to the legislature, for appropriations for salaries, food, and other consumable items. Separate estimates were given for the cost of transporting patients to and from the hospital. In most instances the Assembly granted for operating expenses and transportation the entire sum asked, or close to it. The number of patients increased threefold from 1842 to the eve of the Civil War, from ninety-seven to three hundred. Appropriations rose proportionately, from $16,492.61 for 1842 to about $45,000 for 1859 (the earlier figure included transportation costs, the latter did not, there being a separate sum of $6,000 for transportation).

More white staff was added through the years, including an assistant physician appointed in 1850 to help Galt with the increased number of patients; the staff became more specialized in function, in line with Galt's reform programs. The failure to acquire large tracts of land can be attributed more to disinclination on the part of the administration than to default by the General Assembly. The

Eastern State Hospital's treatment by the assembly in terms of financial support, then, was reasonably adequate, so that the limits of its appropriations may be seen as determined more by the lack of militancy in its leaders (and possibly its declining reputation) than by the parsimony of legislators or governors.

By all accounts Galt had enough means most of the time to fulfill the objective of creating a comfortable and even pleasant physical environment for the patients. There is even a rare extant letter from a patient which speaks of kind treatment and abundant food, albeit plain and deficient in fish and vegetables; she was feeling well enough to go to town to buy a bonnet and veil. The relatively low level of cures probably did reflect, as Galt maintained, the small number of curable cases rather than inadequacies in physical plant or medical care.

Certainly one cannot establish a significant difference in treatment given at the Eastern State Hospital during Galt's administration from that at the more successful mental hospitals in the United States, a few of which had facilities not noticeably better than those of the Williamsburg hospital and which yet reported higher rates of cure. The primary problem at the Williamsburg hospital was that it had to compete with the Staunton hospital, with all the difficulties that that entailed.

CHAPTER FIVE

Administrative Problems and Political Realities 1850-1860

[1]

THOUGH Galt continued the fight with the Western State Hospital for equality in admissions, it seems doubtful that after 1850 he still believed he could match Stribling's accomplishments. Galt did not abandon either moral or medical treatment, but his hopes for therapeutic success were dimmed. Intensifying his discouragement were political and economic problems facing the hospital in the 1850s that adversely affected patients and staff and weakened his already limited administrative authority.

Galt revealed his disillusionment by turning his attention to an entirely new and unorthodox plan for organizing mental hospitals, a plan that he saw as particularly beneficial in dealing with chronic patients. He made his proposals with little expectation of recognition either in Williamsburg or from the psychiatric world at large.

Galt's new scheme, derived from his experience and reading, represented the culmination of much that was best in his thinking about mental illness and was his most significant contribution to that subject. The seeds of the idea, which went beyond the mental hospital to the utilization of an entire community to succor the mentally ill, can be seen early in his career, in his appreciation of the needs of the insane for "normal" surroundings and for continuing contact with sane people. By 1847 he had come to believe that it was "fully as important an indication after a while to separate a maniac from the associations of the hospital as of those at home." Many leading nineteenth-century psychiatrists increasingly approved of and encouraged bringing patients into contact with the sane community through outings and visits, but they did not imply, as Galt's view did, a conviction that the hospital itself at a certain point hindered the patient's recovery.

He rejected the idea of placing mental patients in segregated wards of general hospitals, where the disadvantages of a closed hospital for the insane might be overcome. Sharing his colleagues' indifference to educating the medical profession about insanity, Galt argued that most physicians disliked the insane and would neglect them, and that rich patients in general hospitals would be annoyed and inconvenienced by the special provisions for the insane. No, they had to be in mental hospitals or in a special environment that tried to give them as much of a normal existence as possible.

Finally Galt came up with his new proposal: certain types of patients should be sent to live in the community in a supervised setting. His article "The Farm of St. Anne," published in the *American Journal of Insanity* in 1855, explained his ideas most clearly. He described the employment of patients at the experimental farm of St. Anne at Bicêtre, the famous French mental hospital. Every asylum, he wrote, should likewise have a farm with a house large enough for the farmer, his family, and the farmhands—who would be quiet, chronic patients. The latter would thus enjoy a happier life than in the "crowded wards of an asylum, and also a more useful one," since they would be self-supporting.

Also living on the farm would be "a few lunatics whose unsoundness of mind has not yielded through the operation of various constitutent influences of an asylum; in whom the monotony of an institution seems, indeed, to tally with the character of their derangement, actually giving it a fixedness instead of affording relief." In such patients the same process that had occurred at home was repeated in the hospital: "the patient gradually interweaves his false notions, suspicions and other morbid traits with the constituents of an institution, almost precisely as he had done at home with respect to the circumstances there."

On the farm the patients could enjoy the great benefits of living in a "family circle," without suffering from the harmful associations that their own families would provoke, and would be removed from the impersonal atmosphere pervading most mental hospitals. Further, the undiseased faculties of the mind were more "decidedly" called into play outside the hospital. Another advantage of the plan would be the avoidance of epidemics of sickness that carried off so many inmates in hospital wards, where the sight of dying patients hastened the end of such "weakly constituted persons as the insane." Some chronic disorders seemed to be "aggravated or even engendered by the air itself of a large establishment, contaminated as it is by so many breaths."

The St. Anne system could be improved, Galt suggested, by substituting for the farmhouse a "series of cottages," to house chronic, manageable patients under minimum controls designed more to protect them from the public than the reverse. For some of the less stable nonchronic patients, strong rooms would be required in the central hospital building or in separate cottages. "Indeed," Galt wrote, "I am satisfied that the insane, generally, are susceptible of a much more extended liberty than they are now allowed." In his travels he found some (southern?) institutions superior in this respect to those of New England, which appeared, in contrast, like "prison-houses," notwithstanding their greater comfort and elegance and unsurpassed efficiency. He wished his plan adopted "as much because of the greater degree of liberty which at least [the chronic] insane would attain as for any other reason."

He cited the village of Gheel, Belgium, as superior to American and British hospitals in the management of mental patients. Hundreds of patients exercised in Gheel "nearly the same freedom as the citizens of the commune, going at large everywhere" and living in the homes of the farmers. He quoted approvingly a British commentator who saw in the Gheel system the advantage that the patient's self-respect was not wounded by guards and prison walls: "he feels himself a free man, and instead of being cut off from society, he mingles with his more fortunate fellow-men."

Only by recognizing the prison-like nature of their institutions and adopting such a scheme might American superintendents, Galt declared, "have the honor of establishing at least one new principle in the government of those laboring under mental alienation." Up to that time what had the profession done in this respect? "Absolutely nothing, must be the true answer with every unprejudiced mind." So long as superintendents of the richest asylums devoted themselves to "tinkering with gas-pipes and studying architecture" in order to erect expensive but ugly edifices, no progress in the treatment of insanity in the United States might be expected.

Galt proposed in his annual report for 1854/55 a modified Gheel system for the Eastern State Hospital. An asylum regularly organized and managed according to the true principles of treatment would serve as the nucleus of the community. The hospital itself would be divided into small units where "various feelings of a healthy nature operate." Large assemblages of patients prevented positive feelings and thoughts from developing; they were swamped by the mental disorder all about them. Under his newly proposed scheme the patient would move from a disordering home and environment into a protected situation in the hospital, and then back again by stages into the sane world.

Galt acknowledged that his reorganization plan would not win approval and expected that his ideas would not be implemented. When in 1854 he mentioned the Gheel system at a board meeting, the president told him he should include his plan in the next annual report, which he did then and again the next year, terming such reforms a revolution in the annals of insanity. But, he said, he did not even "attempt to introduce them; neither [was he] wedded to the partial adoption of them now in operation" at the Eastern State Hospital.

The current program of farm work, he pointed out, rather than being a systematic therapeutic device, was a response to requests from local farmers to use patients as laborers. Some chronic patients worked like automatons, with little persuasion, so they were valuable as farmhands. There were also inmates, particularly those only slightly disturbed, who wanted to do farm work for pay. One such, he said, had done so successfully since 1834; another, before his discharge, went out on several trips as a sailor, during which his illness seemed to disappear. A great deal could be accomplished if the insane were not allowed to "sink into solitude and torpor through entire inaction."

One of the sharpest criticisms of Galt's proposals came from Thomas Kirkbride, who was obviously one of Galt's targets in his "Farm of St. Anne" article. Galt could propose such extensive freedom for patients because, Kirkbride said, he had "few but chronic demented cases" and could "have little idea of the restraint really necessary for recent cases, or of the restrictions . . . proper to place on their movements and actions." Those who visited his hospital "know why it is that there is so much liberty permitted between the townpeople and the patients, and which certainly is not seen in any other institution in the country."

Kirkbride's comments were among several rebutting Galt in absentia at the 1855 asylum superintendents' meeting. The participants were, with one or two exceptions, all quite indignant about his remarks on the prison-like atmosphere of New England hospitals and his ridicule of American psychiatrists' contributions to psychiatry. They felt he was receiving his "just deserts" from his critics and that it was too bad the *American Journal of Insanity* should publish "such wholesale slanders."

In 1858 the *Journal* discussed the subject in a review of Galt's latest hospital report. The prominent features of his reform proposals, familiar to the readers of the *Journal*, were

> supplementary erections of a domestic character, near the central institution; the boarding out of selected patients with suitable families; extending to certain others leave of absence on parole, with the view of having them find employment upon adjacent farms, or form other engagements of an analogous character, though still remaining under the treatment and supervision of the superintendent; and a modification of the scheme of "colonization."

Galt's long experience, the editors wrote, entitled his ideas to more serious consideration than the review could give, as did the importance of the subject, his earnestness, and "the fact that similar views have since been as warmly advocated in two leading trans-Atlantic publications." The editors could only say that if any contemporary institution fitted Galt's criticisms, if its inmates were treated as "senseless atoms," subjected to a "daily routine proceeding with the inexorable, monotonous motion of a machine," and invested with "badges of a degrading inferiority," then it was "far behind even the *spirit* of the age." If such a hospital failed to give to each and every patient the greatest freedom his mental condition allowed, the full amount of occupation and amusement his case required, and the associations his comfort and restoration demanded, it had not reached the current standard and did not embody the principles of construction, organization, and management almost unanimously adopted by the American psychiatric profession. "The fault is in the institution and not in the system."

The unsympathetic reception of Galt's views, which were thereby consigned to oblivion, was understandable. He had pushed his own plan at the expense of the reputation of American institutions, almost all of which he deemed inadequate, including by implication some of the best in the North (which he had last visited in 1850). He lauded those (mentioning no names) with no standing, probably the hospital at Baltimore and his own. Then he denigrated American asylum superintendents, a criticism interpreted as not only a back-handed attack on the highly respected Kirkbride, but an insult to men like Luther V. Bell and Isaac Ray who had achieved national and international acknowledgement for their researches and writings.

All this was particularly annoying to members of a young specialty still struggling for public recognition and trying to compete on an equal basis with their European colleagues. The entire psychiatric profession in the United States could easily write Galt off as an armchair critic with views of "very thin Moonshine," who no longer came to association meetings, did not often stir from Williamsburg to visit other hospitals, and had never been to Europe to see psychiatric practices there firsthand. They may also have thought him to be a southern nationalist hostile to New Englanders, especially as they really did not know him well.

Galt developed no close friends in the profession and had not entered fully into the activities of the association, evidently leaving representation from Virginia to Stribling. During the first few years he read a few papers at the association meetings but felt embarrassment at his inability to speak well and anxiety about the social contacts: "At this convention," he wrote in 1849, "I did not remain much in the meeting, purposely avoiding such a source of exposure to dyspepsia—social companionship tends to break in upon habitual observances requisite for our health."

His only real defense at the 1855 meeting came from a Canadian, Dr. Joseph Workman, who praised the people of New England but thought them "rather thin-skinned." The asylum superintendents' own reports, he said, indicated that their institutions "were very far short of perfection," that their architecture had little to recommend it, and that only now were masons tearing down the old strong rooms at the Worcester hospital.

Throughout the controversy Galt insisted on the "ultimate ascendancy" of his program. Soon after the attacks on him at the 1855 association meeting, he wrote a diatribe (in a public letter to the Virginia Senate on the question of the site of a lunatic asylum) against the conformity allegedly demanded by the association's leaders. In all the indignation any merits in Galt's proposals for a cottage-farm and parole system were lost.

After the Civil War, a few concerned persons, among them Dr. Merrick Bemis, superintendent of the Worcester State Hospital, and Dr. Samuel Gridley Howe, reformer and long-time trustee of that institution, advocated the Gheel system but without reference to and probably without knowledge of Galt's ideas. They and later nineteenth-century supporters of the cottage plan accomplished little, indicating that opposition to Galt derived from more than hurt pride and reactions to his hostility. American hospital superintendents were too wedded to their established systems and to the generally accepted view that centralization reduced costs and improved efficiency. "The sooner that *Gheel foolery* is put to rest by the adoption of common sense principles . . . the better for the insane," wrote one superintendent to Kirkbride. "What will do in Holland [*sic*] so far as all experience shows will not do in this country."

[2]

Whatever the theoretical and practical reasons for Galt's scheme to decentralize the hospital, it is difficult not to see its origin also in his own personality and administrative style. The temptation is to draw a parallel between Galt's own expressed need to have contact with people outside the hospital and his insistence that patients would benefit similarly. At the very time he developed this argument for patients he proposed for himself in his diary, "Going into society may affect an invalid by the too great excitement, & the positions of restraint; but familiarity soon gives ease here. And then we have the soothing influences of hilarity & conversation, and the interruption of brooding trains of morbid and introspective thought."

Another time he wrote, "My mind is now so constantly occupied that I have not time for other ideas but those relating to my calling and conversation calls them forth. I am thus led to feel more intensely the want of daily conversation with some stable mind. My fluency would also be thus increased." This observation does not imply that Galt was himself a candidate for a mental hospital; just that perhaps he made use of his personal as well as professional experience and extensive reading to develop his psychiatric ideas.

As an administrator Galt was not strong. He did not have full responsibility for hospital operations, either in principle or in fact, and despite disclaimers was reluctant to take it. To other superintendents who eventually came to know his passivity, he seemed in his decentralization proposals to be trying to reduce their hard-won power to control directly the destiny of the patients. Not that they opposed the participation of laymen in hospital affairs (indeed many wished to increase it), but Galt went too far in seeking to share responsibility for patient care with the community—in boarding out patients, for example.

The old division of authority at the Eastern State Hospital, formal and informal, had been remedied only slightly by the appointment of a medical superintendent. Staff appointments and dismissals remained entirely in the hands of the directors until December 11, 1847, when the board gave the superintendent the same right as a director to nominate the steward and matron and the sole power to appoint all other "subordinate officers." This policy was short-lived. A little more than two years later, on March 23, 1850, the board decided that the right to appoint subordinate officers could not be delegated and withdrew it, leaving to the superintendent the nomination of all the staff but the assistant physician, steward, and matron. The directors could reject or accept his recommendations. All removals remained completely under the authority of the board. The superintendent and the assistant physician would hold office for three-year terms; everyone else would be appointed annually.

That Galt resented this limitation on his authority is evident from his article in the *American Journal of Insanity* soon afterward on the powers of superintendents in mental hospitals. The staff, he wrote, "should be absolutely under his control as to dismissal from their situations; and . . . every such assistant should either be selected by the superintendent immediately, or from his nomination to the board of trustees." The trustees would exercise a check on the superintendent by their right to dismiss him.

Only the superintendent, he declared, thoroughly knew the kind of person needed for each position; the board could not do as good a job of selection. Such bodies, being unpaid and to some extent irresponsible, would not invest the time and energy necessary to make the wisest choices. And by having the superintendent choose his subordinates, responsibility was centralized and successful operation of the hospital promoted, for he could be held to account for the actions of his staff, which would cooperate more effectively with a chief who could fire them. Further, legislative bodies could be sure the "combined advantages of proper treatment and minimum expenditure" would never be fully attained until the superintendent had the control of his subordinates, including their salaries.

Galt advised abolishing the positions of matron and steward, which would mean considerable financial savings. He also favored a consulting physician so that the superintendent might have an outside opinion in doubtful cases and thus assure people that their relatives were receiving proper care. Such a consultant would support the superintendent in the community in countless ways. It was well to have physicians on the board of trustees; they usually helped the superintendent rather than detracted from his power, as might have been supposed.

These and other arguments described Galt's unenviable position at the Eastern State Hospital, especially after 1850 and in contrast with the authority increasingly being granted to superintendents in well-run hospitals. In 1850 he did get as assistant physician his cousin and best friend, Dr. John Williamson, who was selected from among thirty-six candidates; in 1852 the board appointed a second assistant physician to share the work. They were to inspect the wards with Galt two days a week and to alternate daily duty as well, when they administered medicine. This, Galt boasted, the best northern institutions could not duplicate, for they used attendants to give medicine.

But Galt never gained real control over his staff. In 1854 he did oppose, successfully for a time, the appointment of a new matron after the death of Mary A. Galt (for whom the directors ordered a tombstone with an inscription acknowledging her "eminent virtue and invaluable services so long so well and so faithfully performed . . . for forty years"). Even though most medical men would agree on the necessity of a matron, who would live on the premises (unlike Mary Galt, who did not), Galt thought it best to do without. Perhaps this really expressed his resentment of the power the matron had traditionally held at the Eastern State Hospital, a power he could effectively oppose only when the position was vacant. He prevailed only for a while. Six months later the board appointed a new matron, apparently with the understanding that she live within the hospital grounds.

In May 1859 he was authorized to appoint a gatekeeper; a year later the board rescinded this power and reserved it for themselves. The 1852 bylaws stated that the superintendent should "give such instructions and orders to all persons employed at the Asylum, as he shall think proper, and see that they are executed." Lemuel J. Bowden, president of the board, told Galt at a board meeting in 1854 that this meant the superintendent could give any directions he chose to the staff in relation to their duties, as expressed in the bylaws. A reading of the bylaws, however, indicated to the board that this was not so. The directors had undisputed power, but they did not always use it effectively for the better operation of the hospital. At the same time Galt, best situated to do so, lacked the authority to insure compliance of the staff with his directives. The hospital continued, as before, to suffer from ambiguous authority.

Responsibility for this situation lay not entirely with the directors. If Galt had been older when he began and had had a more forceful personality, he probably could have established firmer control over the hospital's internal affairs. For all his complaints, he tended to leave the running of the hospital to others, notably the steward and matron. In 1848 Dorothea Dix raised this question with him after a visit to Williamsburg:

> Your Hospital in all respects but one, disappointed my expectations. . . . I don't think I can be reconciled to the present domestic organization and this all the less from your own non-residence. I think the *Steward* is Superintendent and governor, *not the physician.* This is not well, even supposing him a very excellent person, which certainly I have no reason to doubt. My next objection [is] the non-residence of the Matron, and the third is the evident want of competent attendants and nurses, so far as education and Mental qualifications are considered. These defects, or to me, seeming defects, are not compensated by your assiduity nor by the pleasant location of your Institution.

She liked the good size of the rooms and their neatness, as well as the general air of comfort, but thought there was a "rather . . . prominent tone of *Command*, of *rule*, towards the patients" which might affect them badly. Galt was man enough, she thought, to benefit from her criticisms and accept them in the cordial spirit in which they were offered, without being "wounded thereby."

Miss Dix firmly grasped the situation at the Eastern State Hospital, and it may be that her remarks roused Galt to look more vigorously for better educated white attendants to replace the hired slaves. Yet he continued to live outside the hospital and remained somewhat aloof from its everyday operation, depending very much on the steward to keep him informed and to oversee affairs that did not involve medical judgments. After the assistant physician was appointed Galt noted several times how much more free time he now had to study and pay social calls in comparison with the superintendents of other hospitals. And as he recognized, he was free from the pressure of public opinion in Virginia, where there was not great public interest in the Eastern State Hospital and where he did not have "a variety of state feelings . . . to represent & uphold." "In the want of that intense spirit of progress in Virginia, which is found in other states" he could have more time for study than did other superintendents.

At times he refused to exercise control even when the board gave him the latitude. In the controversy with Stribling over admissions, he abjured any responsibility for decisions over particular patients. True, the boards of both hospitals did have the final authority, as he maintained, but at Staunton one may be sure that Stribling had much to say in the matter. Another instance was typical of Galt's attitude in more petty matters. Various staff officers wanted the hospital's cook to work for them personally; when this was brought to Galt's attention he felt sure that the board would shirk responsibility for the decision and place it on his shoulders—which it did. In principle he did not approve of servants working for the staff and gave all the obvious reasons why they should not. Yet he found it impossible to refuse categorically such a request from his cousin, the daughter of the late matron, Mary Galt.

At another time, when a director said the superintendent should have the power to buy spring clothes for patients and blankets for one who was cold, especially in the steward's absence, Galt denied himself even this small authority. The new board of directors, he explained, "had thought proper to alter the law, in a way not the plan in any other Asylum," which was, however, "immaterial to him." He "had always left to the Steward where he should get purchases" and had "signed bills without having aught to do with their being incurred." It was one thing for Galt to say that he did not handle the purchasing of supplies and that the board had deprived him of this right, but another to insist that even in an emergency he did not have or want the power to buy a blanket for a shivering patient.

Lack of firm centralized administrative authority and the frequent election after 1851 of board members with various personal, pecuniary, and political interests in staff appointments led to constant squabbling among the employees. The controversy between matron Mary Galt and keepers Dickie Galt and Philip Barziza in the 1820s and 1830s was matched in the 1850s by a continuous backbiting that few staff members managed to escape.

Among the many entries in his medical diary noting the infighting over trivial issues Galt mentioned "a very disagreeable scene at the asylum" between two disputants. The argument reached the board, one officer protesting that "charges affecting his character as an officer and his individual honesty have been made against him by another officer . . . in presence of other persons." His request for an investigation was refused because the board had heard no formal charges and had no complaint to make against him. A few months later a director presented a resolution "respecting the duties of officers in being courteous to each other," which touched off a long debate with no results. The rules for tenure of officers must have changed, for it was proposed that annual election of officers would be the only way to make them "behave themselves."

Generally Galt could not bear to hear all the stories of the petty fights and preferred to ignore them or leave their resolution to the board or the steward. "I . . . never interfered in private quarrels," he said. They were all too tedious and disgusting for him; one suspects that he just could not cope with the various personalities and problems, with the result that the patients often suffered. They were used as pawns in the arguments among staff members and were sometimes mistreated, their slave attendants were summoned to work for the staff on hospital time, and the quality and quantity of their food deteriorated at times because of lack of proper supervision.

Once Galt came to the hospital and found "both officers absent," meaning probably the matron and the senior male officer. At another time the whole town of Williamsburg was talking about the latter's threat to knock down an old woman patient who had misbehaved. He claimed that not only was she drunk when she defied his orders but that every day she sent to the female department a bottle of liquor with which which the other patients got drunk. Galt, hearing about the affair from various persons, observed only that he was surprised at the officer's mistreating an old crazy woman and that her husband might learn of it and resent it.

There was also a problem of alcoholism among the staff. In 1856 the night watchman was dismissed for "introducing within the walls of the Asylum ardent spirits and improper company and also . . . causing one of the patients . . . to leave his dormitory & playing on the violin at an improper hour & place." Several years later the board passed a new bylaw prohibiting the "intemperate use of intoxicating spirits by the Officers or men in the Institution" and allowing the discharge of an intoxicated officer or one who on account of the use of ardent spirits became incompetent to perform his duties or who was guilty of any immoral conduct.

It is not clear whether Galt went every day to the hospital during the 1850s. Occasionally he noted in his diary that he must attend more to his asylum duties. At one time he wrote, "Ought I not now to busy myself especially about the Asylum & Asylum matters generally? First because of meeting difficulties at present impending. Secondly I should take advantage of the spirit of improvement in the Directory."

His reluctance to throw himself fully into the running of the hospital was apparent even earlier. The issue was not simply, as he would have it, that heavy administrative duties generally tended to hinder the intellectual activities he cherished so much. Rather, he was not the man to devote himself to administration or to win over, bully, or press the directors to adopt policies or sanction practices that he believed to be in the best interest of the hospital and that the board would not act upon otherwise.

In the case of his Gheel proposals, the Eastern State Hospital missed a chance to be a testing ground for a possibly useful innovation partly because Galt refused to urge its implementation. He tended to retreat from difficult interpersonal or political problems in the hospital; he preferred intellectual pursuits. Though he was supposed to have inspired love, almost adoration, in the patients, he found it difficult to make personal contact with staff officers and felt at a loss when speaking with them.

The large number of incurables was discouraging, but it remained an unsolved problem partly because of Galt's fumbling. Together with the admissions situation and no doubt related to it in some degree, Galt's administrative laxity prevented a more active therapy program at the hospital. During the 1850s life there seems to have gone on monotonously, though not too uncomfortably; the hospital had lapsed into custodialism, the patients left to the ministrations of a lay staff varying in competence and devotion. Galt—reserved, introspective, anxious, gentle, bookish, somewhat hypochondriacal—lacked the leadership qualities usually associated with a good administrator, notwithstanding his considerable intellectual powers, excellent character, and talents as a psychiatrist. Indeed, he appeared rather ineffectual and fearful of exercising authority.

Of course the obstacles were formidable. It was hard for a young man to confront a board whose exercise of almost unlimited powers had precedent behind it of nearly seventy-five years. And once set, the relationship was even harder to change, especially when the directors' pecuniary and personal interests were involved. Between 1851 and 1857 a notably venal board—always involved in some sort of political maneuvering inside and outside the hospital—made Galt's position as superintendent insecure. It may be that he then lost somewhat his commitment to the hospital and chose the path of least resistance in a situation he could do little about.

[3]

In 1850 political developments in Virginia and in Williamsburg brought a change in the government of the Eastern State Hospital. During its earliest years the Court of Directors, recruited from the upper classes of the state, was self-perpetuating and independent of the colonial and state governments. In 1788 the power of appointment went to the governor, but board members continued to serve for life and were usually chosen by incumbents' recommendations from among the "better" families of Williamsburg.

In the 1830s and 1840s this custom brought adherents of the reigning Whig party into office. The board therefore tended to include local dignitaries and politicians, many of them members of successive generations of the same families—Tazewell, Southall, Waller, Saunders, Randolph, Burwell, Cole, Peachy, McCandlish, Griffin, and Galt. At least twenty-two directors served in the state legislature before the Civil War. The long-time president of the board and close friend of the Galts, Robert Saunders, Jr., was at one time professor of mathematics and president pro tem at the College of William and Mary; mayor, magistrate, and councilman of Williamsburg; vestryman of Bruton Parish; and a son-in-law of a governor of Virginia. Others were prominent physicians, professors at the college, lawyers, or merchants from old Williamsburg families.

The situation remained unchallenged at the Eastern State Hospital until 1850, when a change in party alignments brought the Democratic party into power again in Virginia and gave the Democrats a probable majority in the town of Williamsburg. Galt described the effect on the hospital to his uncle in 1852:

> Owing to political differences chiefly, between the Board of Directors of the Asylum, & a portion of the community in the neighborhood, a most harassing contest has been on for a year or two & the affairs of the Asylum have therefore been brought into the arena of politics. This has resulted in a change of the Board of Directors, & several of the officers of the Institution have been displaced.

Before this time, as Galt observed to Stribling, the legislature had done little about Virginia's asylums and perhaps this was for the best; "the less [the superintendent] is at all meddled with by the higher powers, the better."

The leaders of the first organized opposition to the incumbent hospital board were the brothers Lemuel Jackson Bowden and Henry Mosely Bowden. Lemuel Bowden was a prominent and talented lawyer, member of the Virginia legislature from 1841 to 1846 (when he led the fight for the Eastern State Hospital on the territoriality question), delegate to the state constitutional convention, presidential elector in 1860, and during the Civil War a Union senator from Virginia. Henry Bowden was a farmer, contractor, and local politician.

Though from an old family in Williamsburg and James City County, the Bowdens were only recently rich. Lemuel's new house, a handsome, imposing structure said at the time to be the most beautiful in Williamsburg (and still standing next to Bruton Parish Church on Duke of Gloucester Street), was built for him by his brother Henry in 1858 for an alleged sum of $10,000. It testified to the contemporary comment that Lemuel, "decidedly at the head of the bar," was making a fortune.

An early sign of discontent with the government of the Williamsburg hospital was the mention in the December 14, 1849, minutes of the board of a recent article in the pro-Democratic Richmond *Enquirer*, the state's leading newspaper, charging that all the directors were Whigs. The following April Democrats Henry Bowden and D. S. Cowles complained about a dispute with George W. Southall, then a Whig member of the House of Delegates and a hospital director. Southall's insistence, they said, that politics was the issue was only a smoke screen: economics was really at stake, that is, the Eastern State Hospital's unwillingness to pay Bowden and his associates for contracted supplies even after an arbitrator had decided in their favor.

Soon afterwards an open campaign to change the composition of the board was launched. On May 16, 1850, the directors, in electing Williamson assistant physician, created a vacancy on the board. Shortly thereafter a group of prominent Democratic party members from the Williamsburg vicinity, including Henry Bowden, petitioned the Democratic governor, John B. Floyd, to fill the position with an active Democrat, a Williamsburg merchant, John H. Barlow. No incumbent board member voted the Democratic ticket, they said, and it was time the Democratic party received its fair share of representation. In the near future the assembly would surely rectify this situation, as one seat out of eleven on the board would not be enough, considering that the town of Williamsburg had more Democrats than Whigs. The governor should "rescue the Members of the democratic party from a System of proscription which Stigmatises them as a degraded caste for no other reasons than they are democrats." Another letter reminded the governor that all the hospital directors had voted against "us" in the last election. A strong feeling pervaded this controversy that just as white manhood suffrage must become the law of the state, as it did in 1851, so should the white masses gain the rewards of political patronage. Jacksonian Democracy had come to Virginia.

Saunders, the board president, countered the petitions by asking the governor to receive a delegation from the board. This was the first time, he said, that politics had been introduced into hospital affairs, and its influence should be forthwith eliminated. The governor nevertheless appointed Barlow a director.

This was only a first step for the Democrats; the next was to have the legislature change the life tenure of the directors of both the Eastern and Western State hospitals to one or a few years, like that of the directors of the banks and the penitentiary and the visitors of the University of Virginia. Thereafter, the Democrats hoped, the governor would appoint an entirely new slate, mainly Democrats, to run the Eastern State Hospital. At least sixteen or more petitions on the matter, most of them favoring the change and signed by dozens of men from the Williamsburg region, came into the assembly in December 1850, shortly after the recently elected House of Delegates (with many new members) and Senate convened in a new session, with Henry Bowden as the Senate's sergeant-at-arms. The Richmond *Enquirer* again published an editorial critical of the Williamsburg hospital board for being Whig and anti-Democratic.

The hospital directors replied in communications to the Assembly and the *Enquirer* that their opponents' petitions did not reflect public opinion in Virginia. As for the preponderance of Whigs on the board, the legislature must remember that when most of the incumbent directors were appointed, few men in the community other than Whigs would have been proper persons for the positions. Saunders asked, "Why should they [the directors] object to any mode of appointment when their services are performed gratuitously? And, if they desired to use their patronage to further party views, how comes it that of *nine* male salaried officers they should *have appointed six who are Democrats*?" The Democrats answered that the staff might be Democratic, but they voted Whig, and that "those who receive their daily bread from Whig patrons will succumb to Whig influence." Privately Southall admitted, at least to himself, that it "cannot be denied that in this community there is a respectable part of *democrats* here who ought to participate in distributing this patronage."

The issue went beyond mere political patronage. In theory the hospital bought supplies from the lowest bidder. Often enough, however, the low bid did not receive the contract, nor were bids invariably solicited. The steward and other officers sometimes took business where they wished, with no real check on their sources and no contracts. This meant that directors and officers could sell commodities and hire out their slaves to the hospital at will, old practices that made it of considerable advantage to be a director or hospital official, and that continued despite legislative criticisms in 1824 and 1835 and accusations made in 1840 in the press against the directors of both Eastern and Western State hospitals.

All of this created bad feeling among the Williamsburg merchants who did not share in the bounty. At the end of 1850, coinciding with the tenure campaign, Lemuel J. Bowden, Alexander C. Garrett, and Robert H. Armistead preferred charges in writing against the Eastern State Hospital board. After some delay the General Assembly launched an investigation, as requested by the hospital's directors. The Western State Hospital was subjected to a similar inquiry. The clerk of the Williamsburg hospital board wrote Southall that the opposition forces had the votes to remove the present board and that they were "dirty enough to do any thing. Expose them if you can with all of your ability. It can avail nothing with such a body as you have to meet."

The charges against the Eastern State Hospital emphasized economic issues. For example, it was said that in one instance the board gave a contract to supply maize to the hospital to W. W. Vest, its treasurer, and not to the lowest bidder, Jacob Sheldon, a director. The directors replied that since Vest as treasurer received no compensation other than the use of the asylum's money at stated periods, it was "not unfair to any one that he shd be preferred." And although they had raised the rate of return to Vest they "did not think themselves bound to make use of any accidental condition of things, temporarily Existing only to bring down the prices of *Maze* [*sic*] merely for one year, below a fair standard." Further, the evidence showed conclusively that Sheldon's offer "*was nothing more nor less than a bid for the office of treasurer*," so that it would go against the board's public duty "to put up the office of treasurer to the *lowest bidder*. . . ." The bid could not have been accepted anyway, since a board member was not allowed to contract to supply the hospital with goods. The directors denied that the board was packed with Whigs and decried the attempt to make the hospital a "*Party Engine*."

The treasurer, Vest, in correspondence with Southall, evaluated the affair and expressed his contempt for his accusers. Considering the men engaged in the matter and the methods they were using, he would be glad to see the office of treasurer made worthless. Perhaps the legislature might require the annual appropriation to remain in the bank, to be drawn upon only to pay bills as they arose during the year. This would take out of the treasurer's hands the considerable sums of money (never less than ten thousand dollars and very often much more) that he held, sometimes for half a year and more. It might also be best to have the General Assembly choose the hospital's superintendent, and if that proved impossible the governor should do so. Anything rather than have men like Bowden and his friends gain power over the institution. Vest would do everything he could "to cripple the new Directory," even give its powers to the legislature.

The conflict was not only over money and power but also for status; the first two prizes might be won, the last, never:

> I thank God as you do that while they may by a fraud upon the public have everything upset as to the asylum—they still are not on an equality with some others nor can they under any change of circumstances get into that society which next to money they most desire. By every possible means do them all the damage you can—and finally if you fail in hurting them in the lower house—do get Stanard and others in the Senate to fight them to the last. I suppose there never was a case in which more license would be allowed in doing them all manner of harm.

The case for the other side was perhaps most explicitly presented in Barlow's formal deposition and the record of his cross-examination by the Eastern State Hospital directors. To a merchant like himself, he said, the job of hospital treasurer was worth $500 plus $2,000 a year. The first figure comprised the profits realized from the use of the hospitals' legislative appropriations; the second, profits from selling supplies to the hospital. The use of the asylum funds, interest free, was the chief advantage of the office of treasurer, from which the firm of Vest & Co. had profited so well.

Barlow admitted freely that he acted from "considerations of personal interest" in his efforts to reorganize the hospital; he wanted a chance to sell more goods to it. "It was a struggle for power & money . . . between those who are in office & those out." The ins had been there long enough—ten or fifteen years. He did not believe "that the interests & welfare of the institution will be affected one way or the other, either benefitted or injured by the result of the struggle or the proposed change in the Government of the Asylum." Equal representation between Whigs and Democrats could insure that both received fair treatment in the allotment of hospital business.

Jacob Sheldon supported Barlow on the value of the treasurer's office. He noted that although directors were not allowed to engage in contracts with the hospital, nothing was said about whether they should resign before or after making a bid for a contract. Some had resigned after being awarded contracts but before complying with them. "No Director," he said, "would hold the office if thereby excluded from being a bidder."

Whether any official report of the Eastern State Hospital investigation was made is not clear; if, so, it does not seem to have been published. That of the Western State Hospital was. The activities of its treasurer were likewise called into question, and there were charges involving nepotism, irregularities in staff appointments, and irresponsible use of construction funds. The committee saw the evidence, a good deal of it substantiating the accusations, in a light favorable to the Western State Hospital board and to Stribling, who was also implicated. It nevertheless recommended that the hospital adopt a system of accounts less susceptible to corruption, and that the office of treasurer, a sinecure, be eliminated, especially as the hospital's funds were on deposit in a Staunton bank which kept records of their disposition.

After much debate and maneuvering the assembly enacted on March 17, 1851, "An Act changing the mode of Appointment and tenure of office of the directors of the Eastern and Western lunatic asylums." The board of each was to consist of eleven members, their term of office to be three years, beginning November 1, 1851. Five directors were to constitute a quorum, the governor would appoint the new boards and fill all vacancies, and the term of office of the incumbent directors would end on November 1, 1851, or as soon thereafter as their successors were appointed and commissioned.

The funds of the Eastern State Hospital would supposedly be protected by requiring that the treasurer deposit them in a Richmond bank; he could draw money only to meet hospital expenditures and upon the order of the board of directors. Nothing was said about the finances of the Western State Hospital. There was no prohibition against any official or board member having commercial dealings with either hospital, and obviously the office of treasurer was retained. Nor was there any change in the understanding that the directors be local men, which, however convenient for conducting the hospitals' affairs, tended to encourage venality among them.

The method of appointing the superintendent or other hospital officers, another issue in the fight, was not mentioned. Southall, in the debate on the bill, wanted to safeguard Galt's and other jobs by including a provision that no officer could be removed unless by a two-thirds vote of the board. Otherwise he feared that forces hostile to "Dr. Galt, whose eminent qualifications were so well known," would force him out. The opposition denied any such motives and thought the two-thirds principle anti-democratic.

The Democrats had won. The new board of the Eastern State Hospital included Lemuel Bowden, A. C. Garrett, Robert Armistead, and John Barlow. The day they took office Lemuel Bowden was elected president and a new secretary was chosen who had only recently become a Democrat. The next month Barlow became treasurer after resigning as a director; Henry Bowden took his place on the board the following January.

Politics, economics, and social status had become intertwined in this local struggle for power which was in a sense a microcosm of the larger struggles of the time between Whigs and Democrats, ins and outs, old established social classes and a newly rising middle class, rule by elites and more popular distribution of patronage. In Williamsburg, what began ostensibly as a controversy over a contract spilled over into Whig-Democratic politics and enabled the Democratic newcomers to seize control of the hospital that was evidently so lucrative a source of income.

The pre-1851 directors overstated the case in claiming not to ask the politics of prospective staff or board members. They recruited for the board from among their relatives and friends in the upper classes who would naturally be Whigs. No very explicit effort to shut out Democrats was required, just the desire of all established aristocracies, petty or powerful, to choose the "best" men for the enterprises they controlled. And the "best" would be those they knew best. Under such conditions the Democrats and the newly rich (often the same people) would find themselves excluded from the choicest positions such as board membership or the post of treasurer. Representation on the board, probably the most prestigious honorary position in town next to membership on the College of William and Mary's board, would also mean a certain social recognition of the new men. One way to break into the circle was to switch from the economic and social to the political sphere, where the Democrats held power.

Undoubtedly incumbent directors sought to retain their positions for the financial advantages, and not simply for philanthropic purposes, though they were never so bold as the Democrats in admitting this publicly. Throughout much of the Eastern State Hospital's history some directors and staff members, secure in their positions, had benefited financially from their association with the hospital and had appointed friends and relatives to its staff. Just as few, if any, of the directors who served from the end of the Revolution to the end of the Civil War were men of the substance and stature of those named to the first board of 1770, few if not fewer were apparently free of self-serving motives. And there seems to be no record of any outright gift to the hospital by any director subsequent to William Nelson's bequest in 1772 for the maintenance of patients.

[4]

Nevertheless, the pre-1851 directors probably felt a greater obligation to meet the needs of the institution than many of their would-be and actual successors, who were so frank about their economic motives. Certainly the fortunes of the hospital declined during the years the new board was in power, from 1851 to 1857. Nepotism, corruption, and political maneuvering were open and rife; the hospital's operating funds at one time fell dangerously low; and morale and discipline among the staff deteriorated.

Financial manipulations and squabbles, mixed up with politics, soon became apparent. For example, Talbot Sweeney, collector of fees from paying patients, complained to Galt that Colonel Armistead, then a director, moved to reduce Sweeney's percentage because Armistead wanted the job for himself and also because Sweeney had run against him for commonwealth's attorney.

Criticisms of the board reached the newspapers, and by 1855 it was general gossip that all the directors "were pecuniarily interested in the Asylum except two—Mr. [Lemuel] Bowden & Mr. Saunders." One director expressed himself strongly to Galt "against the corruption." During that year the secretary of the commonwealth of Virginia, in a letter to the governor, accused the board, except Saunders, "of being all personally interested in the institution, having contracts" to supply it.

On settling the hospital's accounts, board president Lemuel Bowden said that it "had ten thousand dollars less than he had supposed." Sweeney was accused of getting an "enormous percentage" of profits from supplying the hospital. Most likely the single largest sum taken from the hospital, more than $7,000, went to treasurer Barlow, whose peculation with the pay-patient fund was well known.

At the same time the hospital was suffering, so the board said, from poverty. In 1854 they asked the legislature for more money to compensate for the rise in the prices of goods and the cost of hiring slave labor. The report for 1854/55 also mentioned this problem. In 1855 Barziza, then the hospital's general agent, announced that its depleted funds required changing the patients' diet from wheat bread to corn bread, a plan Galt scotched because it might bring on diarrhea. Whether the difficulty was caused by Barziza's extravagance, as some said, is not clear, but if so, why was there no check on his activities? Another money-saving proposal, reduction of the white staff, was also opposed by Galt. Finally, Barlow said he expressed the board's opinion in suggesting that Galt "should reject all [new] patients, mentioning at the same time that there was a want of funds." The board then ordered Galt, until further notice, to turn away all but paying patients who came from the Eastern State Hospital district and to refuse any, free or paying, from the Western State Hospital.

Meanwhile the hospital's staff as well as its funds was being manipulated, the new board voting some of its members and their friends and relatives into desirable positions. Not only did Henry Bowden become a director but he also hired out slaves to the hospital, and there was talk of his being appointed steward; the incumbent steward, Charles C. P. Waller, for some time felt insecure in his job. Then Henry Bowden's wife, Henrietta Bowden, finally became the matron, after a prolonged struggle and over Galt's opposition to having any matron at all. She was elected on the same day that her brother-in-law Lemuel Bowden, who voted for her, was unanimously re-elected president of the board. The brother, wife, and mother-in-law of yet another board member were appointed to salaried jobs.

In 1852 Dr. Robert M. Garrett, brother of director Alexander Garrett, was appointed an assistant physician at $500 a year, the position being then changed from full-time to half-time, with the right to practice privately as well; the hospital would now have two assistant physicians. Galt's cousin, John Williamson, the first assistant physician, was turned out of his quarters at the hospital and required to give up a third of his salary to the new man and divide his duties with him.

Galt himself was affected. Throughout the controversy of

1850/51 he remained, he said, "pretty much in a neutral position; the Board being a Whig body, & their assailants being democratic." His political principles were "of the latter character." His voting sympathies, however, were often with the Whigs, and he sporadically feared for his job. After the tenure law passed in 1851 he learned from a confidant that Dr. Garrett was rumored to be ready to take his place. It was also said that "Mr. B. . . ." (Bowden?) believed the Galts had had the management of the hospital long enough. Notwithstanding the rumors, the new board reappointed Galt unanimously, to serve at its pleasure.

A little over two years later Galt twice turned down proposals to increase his salary, which had been specified at $1,666.67 in the 1852 bylaws. The first time, early in 1854, he told the board that although he was thankful, he "deemed it inexpedient to raise the supt's salary" to $2,000. Giving Stribling $2,500 had been "one of the most unpopular proceedings that ever occurred" at the Western State Hospital, and Galt feared injury to the Eastern State Hospital if the same were done for him. His close friend Saunders, Galt recorded, whispered to Armistead at the board meeting that he was against the raise lest Dr. Garrett should secure the superintendency.

When the following May the directors, in Galt's absence, voted him an increase to $2,000, he protested again, "because first the supt. should be above the suspicion of grasping at pecuniary matters, and secondly that owing to the crowded state of the medical profession, men with sufficient talent could easily be obtained for the present salary, and for other reasons." In justification of the relatively high pay given him when he first became superintendent Galt noted that at that time "the institution had not been elevated to its present reputation, and therefore medical talent could not be so easily procured." If his salary were now made even more attractive other physicians would find it worthwhile to maneuver for his job, especially since rumors continued about plans to replace him.

The hospital's directors bowed to Galt's wishes and rescinded their order "for reasons assigned by said Superintendent." Stribling evidently had no such qualms (but perhaps also no such problems as Galt). He accepted another raise in 1859 to $3,500 as his just due, telling Dorothea Dix that he had "not the slightest delicacy in taking every cent." He believed that anyone occupying his position earned his salary if he faithfully discharged his duties. Galt on the other hand felt quite noble in his sacrifice, which seemed to him "a fine moral fact" in his "Soul's history." He noted in his diary that the *Saturday Courier* had mentioned his good deed.

By the summer of 1854 he again felt threatened, this time as a result of various machinations in connection with a hotly contested gubernatorial campaign. From then until the following spring the Eastern State Hospital directors and staff were deeply involved in state and local politics. An important issue in that election was the emergence of the Know-Nothings, a nativist party that gained a brief success in 1854 and 1855 in the North by playing on the prejudices of native Americans, especially against Catholic immigrants. In the South, where there were few Catholics, the Know-Nothings attracted support at first because of their equivocal stand on slavery, because they filled a political vacuum left by the dissolution of the Whig party, and because restrictions on immigration would cut down the population of the nonslave North and perhaps quiet the demand for homesteads in free territory. The 1855 spring election in Virginia, preceded by a lively nomination fight the previous fall, aroused great interest and high feelings. The Democrats finally nominated Henry A. Wise, who made very clear his opposition to the Know-Nothings.

For the latter, this first open political struggle was crucial to their fate in the South. In alliance with former Whigs, they nominated what was considered a strong ticket. A Know-Nothing party was formed in Williamsburg, and many staff members and some directors joined. Galt noted in his diary, "Meeting of the Know Nothings . . . Mr. Bowden made a violent speech against the Democratic Party, saying they had gone for a bank man (Mr. Wise) and against the Administration. The Officers of the Asylum were present." (This may have been the beginning of the Bowdens' disaffection with the Democratic party; later they became pro-Unionists and eventually Republicans.)

During the campaign there were various maneuvers and plans to change the personnel of the hospital, including the treasurer and the superintendent, depending on the outcome of the election, with threats on both sides to turn out those who voted "wrong." A Bowden (probably Lemuel Bowden) was said to be after the governorship himself. There were fears that if Wise, a native of Accomack County across Chesapeake Bay, were elected, the present board would be reshuffled, the Bowdens would be out, and Barlow would lose his job as treasurer and have to repay the patients' fund, which would wreck him financially.

Galt wrote in his diary: "Dr. Garrett informed me that since I mentioned a day or two since the project on foot for Peachy (a director) to occupy Sweeney's place [as collector of pay-patients' fees] he had heard further that the whole plan was prepared, based on Wise's election. Mr. Peachy to take the Treasurer's place, Dr. Peachy the Superintendent's &c." Some of the Democratic directors, Galt thought, intended to place him "in the same category with themselves" in order to make it difficult to turn them out without doing the same to him, "& yet to make the odium greater by [his] quietude." Also involved was some sort of religious conflict; evidently the Baptists were fighting for representation at the hospital.

All this insecurity provoked Galt to consider changing his employment. He had speculated in 1851 about all sorts of new careers and interests and then even thought of entering politics himself. In 1852, against his wishes, one wing of the Democratic party ran him for mayor of Williamsburg, and another for magistrate, positions he had refused for years. The results are not clear; according to a letter from his sister he was elected to both, but he did not serve in either post. After a conversation with Henry Bowden at about the same time, he "thought more fully of the advantage upon a close adherence to Party" and his ability thereafter to obtain a job even if he lost his present one. In the first place, his family had "always competed successfully in obtaining popularity." Secondly, the number of public offices was immense and he could get strong recommendations. He really did not want a political career, however, and dreamed about the pleasures of being financially independent with "time to write, to read, to study & for social enjoyments."

Wise won the governorship overwhelmingly, a result that broke the Know-Nothing party in Virginia and signaled its defeat all over the South. It also meant that the anti-Wise men on the Eastern

State Hospital board were finished there for a time, anyway, though Wise could not turn them out until late 1857 when their terms were over. Galt heard that Wise approved of a plan to reform the Eastern State Hospital administration by going out of the Williamsburg neighborhood for better men, reducing the number of directors, and giving the board power to dock salaries or suspend officers.

Wise's victory also gave new heart to the minority opposition on the incumbent board. On March 31, 1856, the directors by a majority of one vote ordered Barlow to draw all money from the state due the hospital as of April 1, but did not require him to deposit it in a Richmond bank, as the law ordered. This was an illegal procedure that enabled the treasurer, as of old, to use the hospital's funds for private business purposes (as Barlow had been doing all along with the pay-patients' fund). In this case the protesting directors stated their case to the state's treasurer; the board rescinded the order a few days later. The real defeat would come when the governor named a new board. Galt wrote at the end of 1856, "Matters at the Asylum are at present in a quiet condition, but as a new Board will be appointed during the next year, I fear we will have to pass through another revolution, and again feel the influence of politics particularly."

But before this could happen Governor Wise tried to make the incumbent directors answer for their activities. In October 1857 he put to the boards of the Eastern and Western State hospitals a series of questions about their administration during 1856 and 1857, including politics and financial transactions. The replies of the Eastern State Hospital directors to the questions about the treasurer's activities revealed a curious attitude of irresponsibility as well as evasiveness. They could not say whether the treasurer's drafts on the state treasury for appropriations were always under the orders of the board. "It is not in our power to say what drafts he has drawn. The auditor must look to that." They believed, however, that they had given him orders on the treasury for all such monies, and if the auditor and state treasurer had helped him to draw money from the state treasury without the board's order, "they alone are culpable and amenable; and sums so drawn would not affect the asylum in any particular." As for various questions on the hospital accounts, there was not enough time to answer all of them; the governor should consult accounts heretofore rendered him.

The board did direct the treasurer to deposit all money drawn from the state treasury in the bank, but there were sums received by him from the pay-patient fund that were needed for current expenses, and it would be "a mockery" of the 1851 law and "not a fair construction" of it to bank such money in Richmond, only to withdraw it "forthwith" and bring it back to Williamsburg to be expended for the uses of the asylum. The board was not aware that any director was personally interested in any contract in relation to the asylum or its support. The directors had sometimes sold marketable commodities to the asylum. "How we should get along without such a course, it is difficult to say" and in any case the sums involved were insignificant.

The board admitted that the treasurer had drawn, on order of April 26, 1856, $7,082.10 from the pay-patient fund. Under a settlement just made he owed the asylum only $2,973.04 out of this sum, only that much being properly applicable to the pay-patient fund. The entire pay-patient fund was needed for "immediate and pressing demands of the asylum," and experience had "shown the absolute necessity of keeping a large amount of [it] constantly on hand to provide for the probable insufficiency in any year of the annual appropriation for support."

The answers of the Western State Hospital board showed a different attitude from that of the Eastern State Hospital directors—but some of the same practices. The administration of the Western State Hospital, both financial and internal, seems to have been governed by more formal and detailed rules and regulations than at the Eastern State Hospital, and the board and the superintendent displayed a good deal more detailed factual knowledge and control over the asylum's affairs than their counterparts at Williamsburg, who appeared to be working on a somewhat informal basis.

The replies further showed the large number of staff members, their families, and their slaves supported by both hospitals. This situation no doubt helped account for the relatively high cost of maintenance per patient and also for the interest taken by politicians and directors in such jobs at the hospital. The saying is, and was, in Williamsburg, that the town was a place where "the lazy take care of the crazy." At the time of the investigation, October 1857, the steward of the Eastern State Hospital lived with his wife and child in five rooms, and his three servants in two rooms, in the Doric building. The ward officer for the Gothic building, his wife, and two nieces had an apartment of three rooms and a closet, and his female slaves lived in an outbuilding. Another ward officer lived in two rooms in the main building, and yet another occupied five rooms there with his wife and four children, his two slaves living in a room in the kitchen.

In four rooms of the center building lived the matron with her husband, three children, and a housekeeper; she also had four servants. The female night watch occupied two rooms with her daughter and a servant girl; the ward officer for female Negro patients lived in two rooms, a "little colored girl" lodging with her at night. Another female ward officer had rooms set aside for her use, as did a third one, who lived there with her two sons and a "little" servant; a fourth ward officer had a storeroom and four rooms for her family, her two slaves occupying a room in the kitchen.

There were also 31 slaves working directly for the hospital, including a male and female cook, a shoemaker, gardener and gas-maker, barber, carriage driver, and jobber. Altogether, the hospital had at least 20 staff members, including 3 physicians; 31 slaves working for the hospital; 17 relatives living with the staff members; 14 slaves belonging to the staff members; and 2 other persons. A minimum of 84 persons, thus, were supported by the hospital, many of them working not for the patients but for the staff and occupying rooms that might otherwise be used for patients. At this time the hospital had 257 patients, so that for about every 3 patients there was 1 staff member, slave, or relative to support. The situation at the Western State Hospital was similar.

Whether affected by the answers to his questions or not—it is hard to think he was not—the governor shortly thereafter replaced the Eastern State Hospital board by men of his own choosing. Barlow, of course, lost his job as treasurer. Notwithstanding the board's manipulation of the figures, he owed the hospital $7,393.61. A "Communication Relative to the Pay Patient Fund of the Eastern Lunatic Asylum, 1857–58" addressed to the General Assembly at its request by the new president of the board declared that Barlow was indebted to the hospital for $5,152.61 from the pay-patient fund and for another sum of $2,241.00, the balance of a special appropriation made during the session of 1855/56 for repairs and purchase of furniture. He could not and would not repay the money, despite efforts to get him to; at least before the Civil War he did not pay, if ever.

The new board, serving from 1857 to 1860, boasted of reducing costs and bringing the hospital to a prosperous condition. On taking office they told the General Assembly they "found a great deficiency in the clothing of the patients and in the various articles of furniture needed for their comfort, such as bedding, bed clothes, and chamber and dining room furniture." The buildings needed repair, as did the drainage and sewerage of the entire institution. The hospital was "destitute not only of the comforts, but also of the common necessaries of life. Every ward and every department was deficient in proper appliances," all showing signs of gross neglect.

Under the new board the exteriors of the buildings were refurbished and new roofing installed; the interiors were repaired, painted, and plastered; and the exterior wall was mended. All this and more was accomplished without going beyond the general funds for the hospital's support from 1858 to 1860. The families of officers were removed from the hospital, making room for more patients, on whom the board now spent an average of only $178.94 a year as compared with the $251.93 of their predecessors. The previous hospital officers were investigated and minor changes in procedures made. Most important, the directors prohibited themselves or any officer connected with the asylum from supplying it; they maintained, too, that they did not give rewarding jobs to their relatives.

These last reforms came rather late, in fact not until a few months before another investigation by the governor in October of 1860. Hence, it seems that the profits to be gained through association with the hospital were practically irresistible, whatever the political complexion of the board. The governor inquired into the interests of directors in contracts for the asylum and into charges of nepotism, particularly concerning the job of clerk-storekeeper held by the son of a director.

The board replied that if there was an understanding between the present meat supplier and the former one, now a director, the board, though believing there was nothing of the kind, considered that they had nothing to do with the case. Their reply to the governor also showed that W. W. Vest had returned as an agent for the board to buy groceries, medicine, clothing, and other goods for the hospital and that medicines had been bought from two directors until 1859 and 1860. But in February 1860 the board "Ordered that from this date no supplies of any kind for the use of the Asylum be purchased from or forwarded by any member of the Board of Directors or any officer connected with the Institution." The board concluded its answer with a statement of the nepotism of its predecessors. As for the appointment of the clerk and storekeeper under its administration, the father and son denied any favoritism or prior agreements; the father did not vote for the son, he said, nor did he use his influence to have him appointed.

What happened at the Eastern State Hospital during the 1850s was not unique. Similar instances of political influence, patronage, and corruption troubled other state hospitals, where sometimes superintendents' appointments were blatantly political and whole hospital staffs were displaced after state elections. And with Governor Wise's accession and the appointment of a new, somewhat less venal and more conscientious board, the problem was not over for the Eastern State Hospital. Not only did the new directors also tend to look for pecuniary advantages, but also the law concerning appointments was kept on the books, so that whatever the institution accomplished it must always reckon with the political powers and local worthies that wanted to use it as a patronage plum. In 1858, for example, Galt again felt his position shaky and tried to prepare himself for the worst. The days of relative immunity from political interference ended in 1850. From that time on, the hospital was seldom free of the vicissitudes of politics, a situation that became even more acute during the turbulent Civil War and Reconstruction years.

That the politics and patronage of the 1850s affected the patients adversely is clear, and not only through creating deficiencies in food, clothing, and upkeep of buildings and grounds. Equally deleterious were the lowered staff morale and weak administration, especially obvious in Galt's reduced interest in hospital affairs. At the least, the political conflicts must have contributed to the lowering of the hospital's reputation and to the erosion of the atmosphere of hope and confidence so necessary to a hospital that sought to be more than merely custodial. Whatever the intensity and effects of the various controversies involving the hospital during the decade or so before the war, however, they fell into insignificance in comparison with the national crisis of the 1860s, from whose influence not even a small, sleepy little institution for the insane would be exempt.

KEY TO FIGURE 9

A.	Public Hospital	Built 1770 3rd story added 1838-1840 Burned 1885
B.	East Building	Built ca. 1820 Enlarged 1833-1835 Burned 1885
C.	Convalescent House	Built before 1821 Torn down ca. 1855
D.	West Building	Built 1824-1826 Enlarged 1833-1835 Burned 1885
E.	West Wing	Built 1838-1840 Burned 1885
F.	East Wing	Built 1843-1845 Burned 1885
G.	Wood Verandahs	Built ca. 1845 Torn down 1885
H.	Gothic Building	Built ca. 1848-1850 Enlarged ca. 1883 Burned 1902
J.	Doric Building	Built 1850 Burned 1885
K.	West Covered Way	Built 1850 Burned 1885
L.	Chapel	Built 1869-1872 Burned 1876
M.	East Covered Way	Built 1869-1872 Burned 1876
N.	Jacobean Building	Built 1869-1872 Burned 1885
O.	Outbuildings	
P.	Galt Cottage	18th C. with later additions; moved—now on Tyler St.

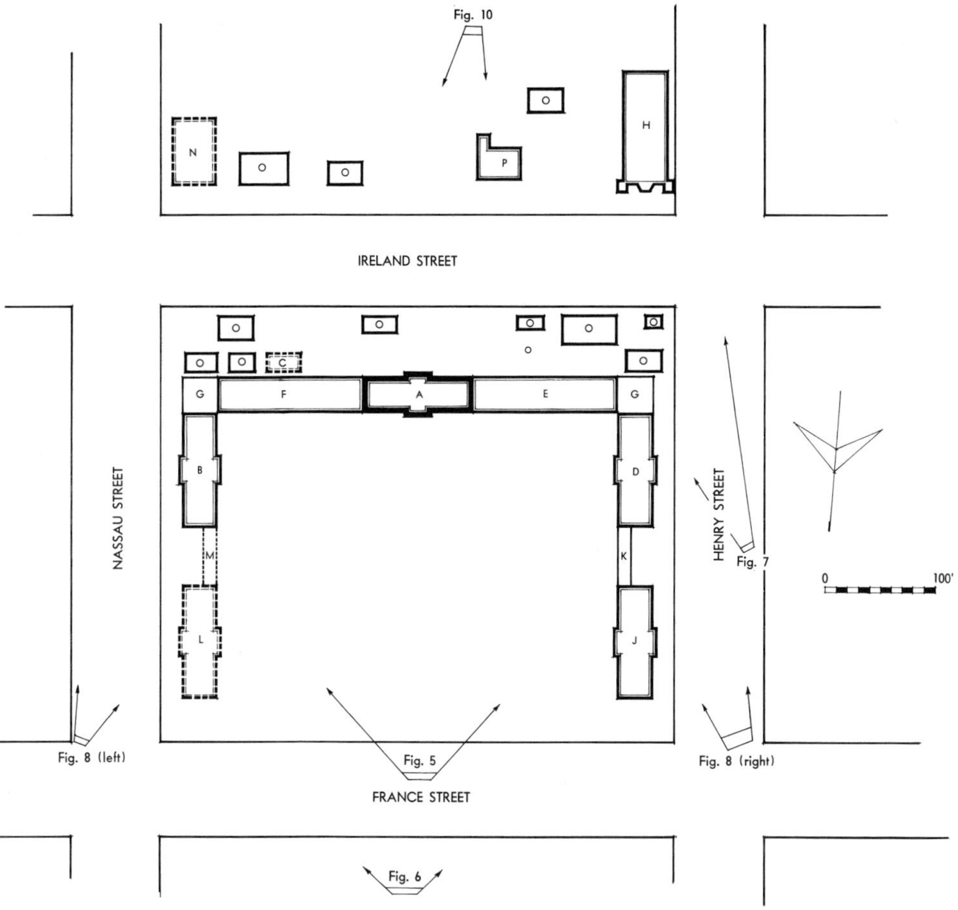

Figure 9
Conjectural Site Plan

In this 1970 drawing all major and some minor hospital buildings up to about 1885 are shown as surviving documentary evidence seems to place them. At least one (not including outbuildings) had been torn down by about 1855, and others were not built until 1869. Points of view of other illustrations in this book are indicated.

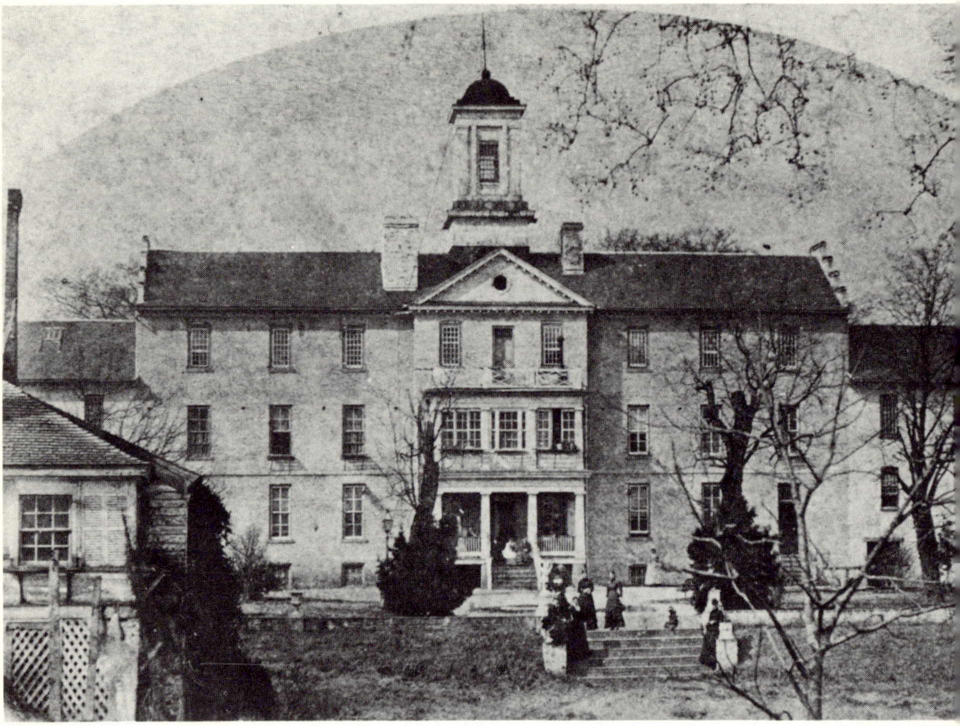

Figure 10
Main Building of the Hospital from the South

A photograph taken before fire destroyed the building in 1885. The third story had been added about 1840. A corner of the "Galt Cottage" appears in the left foreground.

CHAPTER SIX

The War and Afterward
1861-1866

[1]

THE Eastern State Hospital faced the war years with a new board and a new name. The name lasted a long time, the board but little more than a year. At the end of 1860 the three-year term of the 1857 directors was over and new members were appointed, the former president, Robert Saunders, among them. The following March 26 the legislature changed the name of the Williamsburg hospital to Eastern Lunatic Asylum; the Staunton hospital was called Central Lunatic Asylum, and the new hospital beyond the mountains at Weston, the Northwestern Lunatic Asylum. A few weeks later came the firing on Fort Sumter, Lincoln's call to arms, Virginia's secession from the Union, and the designation of Richmond as capital of the Confederate States of America. Virginia became a major battlefield of the war and Williamsburg a minor outpost.

Almost from the beginning there were troop movements through Williamsburg. It lay on the road between Richmond and Fort Monroe, the Union stronghold at the tip of the peninsula formed by the James and York rivers. The ladies of the town, including Galt's sister Sally, were kept busy making beds for hospitals being prepared in expectation of battles in southeastern Virginia. Several officers stayed with the Galts, and about a thousand soldiers visited the hospital during the spring of 1861. One noted in his journal that Williamsburg, "an ancient and decayed town," had one of the state's two lunatic asylums—it seemed strange to him that Virginia should need more than one—" a very large and imposing building," but there was "nothing beautiful about it." In the fall of that year all the churches in town were used as Confederate hospitals, so that the Methodist, Baptist, and Episcopal ministers had to preach in the chapel at the asylum. Until the evacuation of Williamsburg by the Confederates in May 1862 the Galts housed sick Confederate soldiers; Sally Galt also sent food to those in the improvised hospitals and considered herself their "Patron Saint."

By the end of 1861 prices had risen so high that the hospital board petitioned the legislature to grant it $60,000 for the next year instead of the $45,000 appropriated the previous year. They received only $45,000 (as did the Western State Hospital) plus $3,000 for patients' transportation and an additional $10,187 out of the unexpended balance from the year before.

Really hard days for the hospital came with the Peninsular campaign of 1862. Williamsburg lay in the line of march of McClellan's Army of the Potomac, massing at Fort Monroe to advance up the peninsula against Richmond. Situated on a land rise between the York and James rivers, the town was a natural point of Confederate defense. While the siege and battle of Yorktown delayed McClellan's army the Confederates feverishly shored up their lines two miles below Williamsburg. These fortifications, known as Fort Magruder, served as the chief defense of the region. General Joseph E. Johnston, commander of the Confederate army, made the mansion of W. W. Vest, Eastern State Hospital's former treasurer and current agent, his headquarters. Vest, along with most if not all of the hospital's directors and other prominent Williamsburg citizens, had fled in expectation of a Union invasion. Saunders was given the right to conduct all the hospital's affairs, but he also soon left. The last board meeting recorded during the war was on the final day of April 1862.

On May 5, a rainy day, the expected battle—really a skirmish—took place outside Williamsburg. The women gave food to the Confederates passing through, and some citizens walked out, umbrellas over their heads their only protection, to observe the fighting; others watched from the Gothic tower of the Eastern State Hospital, which was not only safer but offered a clear view of the neighborhood. Each side claimed a victory, but that night the Confederates evacuated Williamsburg.

The next morning the Union soldiers followed them in, McClellan replacing Johnston at the Vest house, which was used as a Union headquarters throughout the occupation. One resident recalled the magnificent sight of "countless thousands of blue-clad troops, all in new uniforms" passing through Williamsburg. The town was filled with the wounded of both sides, who were treated impartially by Dr. R. M. Garrett, then consulting physician to the Eastern State Hospital and "a strong Southern sympathizer." The College of William and Mary, used by both armies in turn as barracks, hospitals, and offices, stored most of its "Philosophical Apparatus" at Eastern State, along with the marble statue of Lord Botetourt, one-time royal governor of colonial Virginia; later, books saved from the college fire of 1862 were taken there.

On May 10 McClellan moved northwest, leaving Williamsburg under the control of the Fifth Pennsylvania Cavalry; the regimental commander, Colonel David Campbell, was appointed military governor and then provost marshal. The town was thereby placed under martial law and governed by a Union provost marshal throughout the war. It was, however, never securely held by the Union forces but served rather as an outpost, patrolled by pickets from Fort Magruder and frequently attacked by small groups of Confederate cavalry. Though no longer important militarily, it remained significant as a center of military intelligence and communication. For nearly two years the Williamsburg area was the closest Union position to Richmond. One Union officer recorded:

> In consequence, it became . . . a salient point of observation in the whole military line drawn about the Confederacy; a principal channel in securing the latest news from the Southern capital, sometimes of great value to the War Dept. at Washington, with which it was connected by telegraph lines starting from Fort Magruder. It was an important terminal for the

> arrival and departure of spies in the employ of the Department, as well as for scouts belonging to commands within [Union] lines.

The Confederates also used Williamsburg, whose citizens were strongly pro-Confederate, as a valuable source of news and a mailing station connecting them with the outside world. Because of the town's situation and also because he was a volunteer officer of staunch Unionist (and anti-Rebel) sympathies, Provost Marshal Campbell showed little restraint in using the powers that made him, "within the city's precincts, practically an autocrat."

Shortly after the entry of Federal troops John M. Galt II died. An obituary described the event: "Died, in Williamsburg, Va., May 18th, 1862, after an illness of four days, of an affection of the stomach, to which he had been subject for many years, and which reflecting on the brain, caused apoplexy. . . ."A distant cousin, writing in 1900, related the following: "When in May, 1862, the Union troops took possession of the town and hospital and he was not allowed to enter the hospital, his anxiety about the patients was so great that he could neither eat nor sleep for several days and nights, and it is thought that this caused his death." The source of this interpretation is not given, but recent writers have repeated the story, adding, also with no documentation, that a Union soldier with a fixed bayonet barred Galt's way.

From the contemporary evidence examined, all one can know is that Galt died on either May 17 or 18, less than two weeks after Williamsburg fell into Federal hands. A fragment of a biographical sketch of him, written possibly by his cousin and in the handwriting of his sister Sally (who may have written the obituary or furnished information for it), says, "Though robust in appearance the physical health of Dr. Galt was not good, & 'singularly temperate in all things' he was yet for many years subject to dyspepsia. In the midst of his philanthropic labors fatal disease came . . . & after four days illness he died on the 17th of May 1862."

Sally Galt may have forgotten the exact date, which seems unlikely; certainly she would not have forgotten the circumstances or forgiven any Union responsibility for her adored brother's death.

In none of her other extant letters and documents preserved at Williamsburg did she mention that he was prevented from entering the hospital, even though she commented later that secessionist feeling was so fierce in Williamsburg and spying so rife that the Yankees had to be strict with the residents.

A few months after John M. Galt's death, Dr. John Galt Williamson, his cousin and closest friend and the hospital's assistant physician, also died. Sally Galt recalled that he told her "he could not survive John & his words proved prophetic." So ended the official connection of the Galt family with the Eastern State Hospital after almost a century of devotion to the insane.

Only forty-three years old when he died, John M. Galt II had served the hospital faithfully for twenty-one years, all his adult life. Though not able to raise the hospital to first rank among American mental institutions, he did lift it from provincial doldrums to modernity, as understood in his day. He brought to the patients a warm, understanding sympathy and concern for their condition. In psychiatric theory he was something of an innovator; there lay some of his greatest talents and best inclinations.

How much further he would have gone in his thinking had he lived longer is of course unknown. Some men mature quickly and do their most important work early; Galt's intellectual activity did not follow that pattern. He had a skeptical and inquiring outlook, consciously flexible, eclectic, and committed to change and the value of scientific investigation. With increased experience and knowledge his views changed, and he developed some of his best ideas during his middle and late thirties, so that it may well be that death kept him from making his most valuable contributions to psychiatry. In his lifetime he did not gain the recognition he so much wanted, and it is doubtful that he could have.

Despite his conscientious and varied intellectual work, Galt never became as prominent and respected as did Amariah Brigham, Isaac Ray, and Samuel B. Woodward in the North—asylum superintendents known to the educated public and in touch with leading lawyers, reformers, and intellectuals—nor even as successful as the practical administrator Francis Stribling. Galt's ideas on hospital organization diverged too sharply from psychiatric thought then and for generations thereafter, and his disillusionment and self-imposed isolation helped eventually to alienate his colleagues from him.

It is unlikely that had Galt survived he would have done well in competing for state legislative favor or funds in the political scrambles of the war and postwar periods. Possibly he would have continued as superintendent throughout the war, whether he took the oath of allegiance to the federal government or not. If so, the patients would have had an experienced physician instead of the various inexperienced, temporary chiefs who served during the turmoil of the war and afterward. Any projection of what might or might not have happened to the Eastern State Hospital involves the question raised by one writer of "why Federal authorities chose to take over a civilian mental hospital by force of arms. Had Dr. Galt been permitted to continue his duties, it would have saved valuable military personnel for other duties."

[2]

In the first place, it is not at all certain that the military authorities took over the hospital before Galt's death and by force of arms. The available evidence indicates that they stepped in to save the hospital, stepped out when a civilian superintendent appeared on the scene, and came back when the hospital again lost its civilian supervision.

With the superintendent dead and all the directors having fled Williamsburg, the hospital had no leadership, and certainly the Union command could not have been expected to apply to Richmond for a new superintendent or board of directors. Apparently toward the end of May the Federals appointed a military surgeon to take charge, a Dr. W. Clinton Thompson. A contemporary diarist, Miss Harriette Cary, writing on May 26, observed, "Since Dr. Galt's death a Yankee has been appointed his successor which was but the beginning of a complete revolution in the Asylum government—with the exception of steward and one of the inferior officers, who have been retained for some reason." The next day she wrote, "The officers at the Asylum have not as yet been superseded but have received orders, and are making preparations to leave—the Bowdens are supreme and will exercise authority over the institution hereafter." Henry Bowden later testified that on May 26 he was appointed clerk, replacing Charles Waller (formerly the steward), then away visiting his sick child.

Provost Marshal Campbell may have preferred to have one of his own men in charge. It may also be that immediately after Galt died some staff members were deposed and others more friendly to the Union installed in their places, as the Confederates believed. There seems to be no evidence that Campbell or his superiors considered the asylum a refuge for southern spies and the like and so wanted it under their control, but they might have. Seemingly an innocent haven for refugees and for valuables, as well as the insane, it could have become a clandestine Confederate intelligence center. In October 1862, for example, Talbot Sweeney, terming himself the "deposed but rightful attorney" for the Eastern State Hospital, included in a letter to Governor Letcher describing the hospital's condition some military intelligence for the governor's information.

As for the Bowdens, Miss Cary recorded on May 12 that "Bowden, the Traitor" was mayor of Williamsburg. This probably was Lemuel Bowden. He was such a strong Unionist that his mother, an "ardent secessionist," a memoir recalls, refused to live in his elegant new house. It was probably true that the brothers, earlier so closely associated with the hospital, wanted to purge it of secessionist sympathizers—of whom there were many, including the Galts—and to take over their posts. And in a short time not only Henry but his wife Henrietta and his nephew Thomas R. Bowden were installed at the hospital.

Lemuel Bowden thought that even the strict Campbell was too lenient with the Confederates. He later demanded that Campbell be replaced with a man strong enough to restore Unionists to their homes and that the "Letcher and Davis men appointed by Campbell to office, be removed." (This last may have referred in part to the staff members appointed by Campbell to run the asylum when the Bowdens and their friends left in August.)

Meanwhile, the General Assembly in Confederate Richmond was

concerned about the hospital, "fallen into the possession of the enemy," its "unfortunate inmates . . . incapable of taking care of themselves, or of making known their wants and sufferings," and who were or might be "deprived of the care and control of their natural friends and guardians." On May 17 Governor Letcher was authorized to appoint one or more persons to visit the hospital, if the Union command allowed it, and upon the report of the investigators "to adopt such measures as may be in his power for the preservation of the institution and the care and comfort of its patients, and to use for that purpose the funds appropriated for the institution, or if required, the contingent fund."

McClellan gave permission for the mission, and Letcher selected Judge W. W. Crump and Confederate surgeon Dr. St. George Peachy, of the Peachy family of Williamsburg, to go to the Eastern State Hospital through the Union lines, then occupying the whole peninsula from outside Richmond to Fort Monroe. Peachy, needed at Richmond, did not go, so that Crump, who seemed to know everyone in power on both sides, started out alone on May 26 under a flag of truce. His daughter recalled the trip years later: On arriving at Williamsburg, he found that the asylum "had been taken charge of by Col. Campbell and everything in good condition, they having command of much greater means than our Governor; after going through and seeing everything in most satisfactory condition he felt more than content to leave it in their hands."

During this time it seems that pro-Union Virginians (possibly including the Bowdens) in contact with the Unionist state government in Wheeling were trying to take over the hospital in the name of that government. The choice made by Governor Francis Pierpont (also called Pierpoint) for superintendent was Dr. Gillet F. Watson, a physician and politician from the Eastern Shore of Virginia about whom little is known. Campbell would not give up the hospital to Watson without authority, so Watson went to Union headquarters on the peninsula to see the commanding general. Succeeding in his mission, he took charge of the Eastern State Hospital on June 5, under authority of General McClellan and under appointment of Governor Pierpont, "with full powers to manage the same until a loyal board of directors be appointed."

Watson "found the Physicians and officers extreme Rebels . . . and made a clear discharge of them all." Under instructions from Pierpont he required the staff to take the oath of allegiance to the United States of America. "Henry M. Bowden, Summerset [*sic*] Moore, Jno. W. Hutchings, Thomas R. Bowden, Robert Bachan, Felix Logue, John Bacon, and Henrietta S. Bowden" took the oath. Refusing were "Doct. John G. Williamson, Doct. Robert M. Garrett, William R. C. Douglas, R. R. A. Bowry, Allen Lindsay, William Goodman, Elizabeth Ware, Elizabeth C. Ware, Sarah Roper and Mary Roper, and also Mrs. Jane Moore." Watson appointed Henry Bowden to be steward in Douglas's place, and since all the staff physicians were now gone, obtained permission from McClellan to have Dr. Thompson, the military surgeon, remain as his assistant.

Watson discovered more to criticize at the hospital than had Judge Crump. When Dr. Thompson took charge, the patients were suffering from a scarcity of provisions. Apparently expecting the civilian authorities to take over soon, he did not lay up a store of supplies. Watson reported to Pierpont that the hospital lacked clothing, medicines, and provisions of any consequence, and so he went to Philadelphia to buy them: "The expenditure of the institution for the past year was $60,000. I hope to do your appointment honor. I think I can supply every want and comfort for $40,000. My aim will be to build up the institution. There is much room for improvement. I would like you would pay it a visit when I have had time to arrange matters."

Dr. Watson's ambitions were disappointed; his term of office lasted only a little more than two months, though his salary as superintendent seems to have continued beyond then. In August McClellan, his attempt to take Richmond unsuccessful, was in full retreat down the peninsula with an army that "didn't look so splendid then." The town was faced with evacuation of the Union forces, and Watson, Henry Bowden and his family, and other Union sympathizers within and without the hospital prepared to leave. On August 20 Watson telegraphed President Lincoln:

I am senator of the Wheeling Government & under Gov.

> Pierepoint [*sic*] appointment am Supt. of the Eastern Lunatic Asylum. Williamsburg is being evacuated by the Union forces. Under these circumstances the safety of my life requires that I shall leave in a very few hours—When I leave all the officers and servants will leave so that the Unfortunate inmates will be left locked up without any one to minister unto them. I have made known this condition of things to Genl Dix and Genl McClellan and they have done nothing! I now communicate it to you which is the last effort—I can make—

After the war there was some controversy and an investigation into the circumstances of Watson's and Bowden's departure, they being accused of carrying off the asylum's provisions with them, leaving the patients destitute of food, clothing, supplies, and furniture, and of mutilating and taking official records. Henry Bowden testified that they took the supplies on orders from President Lincoln in reply to Watson's telegram. Lincoln told them, he said, to "leave the institution, take care of your officers, and leave nothing that you carried there." Whether Lincoln did send such a message it is difficult if not impossible to discover. There was also a question of the mysterious disappearance of $12,000 drawn from the Virginia state treasury for the Eastern State Hospital in May 1862 and of the record of the transaction. Watson's military successor as superintendent testified that Watson told him he had spent half the money supplying the hospital, but apparently no other information about it came to light.

In any case, the hospital was left in bad shape. The 252 patients had but one white staff member, Somersett Moore, a ward master, to oversee their care and only enough food for supper that night of August 20. The Union army, still in the area, came to the rescue. Moore delivered the hospital keys to Colonel Campbell, told him of the patients' plight, and was thereupon requested to remain as clerk and take charge. The next day the army began to supply the hospital with stores. The local commander appointed as superintendent Dr. Peter Wager, an assistant surgeon of the Fifth Pennsylvania Cavalry who had visited the hospital several times when it was under Watson. He also asked the former deposed officers (who had refused the oath) to return to work, with no conditions. Campbell told the commanding general, "The patients will be properly cared for" and wired Watson that he supplied the asylum with "thirty days ration & sent back the old officers. All quiet here."

The Federals, still holding Williamsburg, continued to supply the hospital, run by Wager and the former staff. In October 1862 Governor Letcher in Richmond, concerned again about the "distressing reports as to the conditions of the lunatics," and unable to get reliable information, wanted to send Colonel Benjamin S. Ewell, former president of the College of William and Mary, and James W. Custis of the House of Delegates to investigate, but they were refused passage through the Federal lines. Letcher protested this in his annual message "as a scandalous outrage upon the principles of civilization and the dictates of christian [*sic*] humanity."

He received information about the hospital a few days later from Talbot Sweeney, who said the patients had enough to eat, "*such as it is*," but lacked clothing and "attention of every kind." For the last ten days they had received no medical treatment because the superintendent had gone to Philadelphia and left no one to take his place. Nor was this the only time that patients had no medical attention since the Federals took over the hospital. The slave servants hired at the beginning of the year took their freedom, and those remaining were under no restraint and indifferent to the patients' needs. They were ever alert to leave if the Confederate armies approached. The Union staff members at the hospital had run away at the first sign of danger while the Confederate sympathizers "without a single exception" had met the Federals firmly and without servility. After the "stampede" of the Union men, Colonel Campbell,

> finding himself in a sad predicament, invited the old officers to return to their several posts, with one or two exceptions, without accompanying his invitation with the condition of the *hateful parole or oath*. The steward and matron, from what they considered a sense of duty to the patients, there being no one to attend to them, . . . moved back to the Institution.

The rest of the staff went there during the day, Sweeney continued, but none had his heart in the work, the inmates suffered, and the mortality rate was high. If the governor or the president of the asylum, Robert Saunders (who must have been in Richmond), could say that they would not consider it a compromise of their rightful authority over the institution or of the staff's personal honor to do so, the staff "would all return with a good will and do all in their power under existing circumstances to ameliorate the present unhappy condition of the inmates."

There were rumors, Sweeney reported, that the Union army would send the inmates north and use the hospital buildings as barracks. Its own appointees had fled, "and no loyal citizen of Virginia" would accept an appointment from the enemy, so that there might be truth in the talk. Such a course, if followed by the Federals, would probably spell the eventual destruction of the institution by fire. The governor's assurance that the staff could legitimately work under Federal auspices would remove one inducement to the dispersal of patients.

Another problem was that the staff had worked without pay for half a year. They would not take money from the Federal government, and Confederate currency, which was not accepted by the Federals, went at a 50 percent discount in Confederate transactions. Sweeney asked Letcher to send the required funds, which he would distribute. The staff knew nothing of his proposals, nor must the Federal authorities learn of them. Saunders would vouch for Sweeney's integrity.

The reappointed steward of the hospital, Douglas, also complained to Letcher about the lack of slave servants; without them little could be done at the hospital. The few remaining would leave during the Christmas holidays. Nor had the Federal forces yet supplied sufficient fuel, although they distributed enough food and clothing for the winter.

Two discharged patients who made their way to Richmond told Letcher that the "medical attendants were faithful and attentive, and they believed were well qualified for their positions." Supplies for patients were ample but badly prepared, "owing to the difficulty of controlling the servants." These former patients had to get to Richmond as best they could, without funds or provisions; Letcher gave them money to return to their homes.

In March 1863 the General Assembly, despite the Union possession of the hospital, appropriated $48,000 "for support (in addition to the pay-patient fund) and transportation of patients to the Eastern Lunatic Asylum," plus funds to be paid to Saunders and Edward H. Lively for the hire of their slaves for 1862 and to an officer for services in 1862.

[3]

The asylum would soon be in Confederate hands. Rebel guerrillas under command of General Wise, the former governor, who knew the area well, continually plagued the town with sniping and sudden raids. On September 9, 1862, Wise (to punish Campbell for having civilian secessionists imprisoned, albeit they were soon released by his more lenient superiors) had Campbell kidnapped and treated as a prisoner of war.

Partly in retaliation, a few men from the Fifth Pennsylvania Cavalry burned the College of William and Mary the day Campbell was taken, and later his successor closed Bruton Parish Church because of "disloyal utterances" in the pulpit. That winter Wise's troops, probably wanting revenge in turn, continued to raid Williamsburg and at the end of March tried unsuccessfully to capture Fort Magruder, helped by information from the townspeople, including Eastern State Hospital steward Douglas, watching from the hospital's tower. Following this attempt, the Federals placed strict limits on the movements of Williamsburg residents.

The final raid, one that had severe consequences for the hospital, came on April 11, when everyone from the vicinity took refuge there. This time Wise was more successful; though he did not capture Fort Magruder, he drove the Federals out of Williamsburg and occupied it for a few days. He thereby came into possession of the hospital, a situation he did not at all relish for his troops had no resources to run it. To avoid re-enslavement, most of the former slaves ran away, as did practically all the civilian staff; many of the latter, Confederate sympathizers, were apparently encouraged to leave by the raiders. As Saunders later testified, "In the uncertainty, confusion, and excitement of the moment all the superior officers connected with the asylum (who had been appointed by the board) left town except Talbot Sweeney."

Wager, the Union army surgeon in charge, and the two cavalrymen detailed to work at the asylum as attendants were apparently captured by Wise's troops and paroled to work at the asylum, but their position was not clear. Wager immediately approached Wise about what was to be done with the hospital, and two days later wrote Wise that it lacked provisions and fuel and that the Confederates had taken his horse and some of the servants. Should he consider himself a paroled prisoner of war, Wager asked, and would his personal property, especially his horse, be respected? This letter placed General Wise in an embarrassing position, for he did not want responsibility for the hospital (especially as he did not intend to occupy the town permanently, a fact he could not disclose to Wager).

Wise therefore responded that he had no intention of interfering with the hospital and Wager would receive every consideration necessary to the proper discharge of his duties. He was not a prisoner of war, but he and his staff would be bound by parole of honor not to divulge military information harmful to the Confederates. His personal effects would be respected, especially as he was so kind to the patients and the people generally, and the right to bring in supplies from the Union army would be guaranteed.

Nothing was said about the Confederates carrying off, along with former slaves, the hospital's provisions, including medical supplies, as reported by a Union memoirist, who commented "Evidently, the Rebels cared no more for lunatics than the Yankees cared for Collegians; and men of the Fifth hurled back the charge of 'barbarity.'" Wise himself, in a letter to his superior, reported that his forces had gathered "all the plunder we could find [in the town] and [moved] out the inhabitants and their effects."

Conditions at the hospital became desperate. Sally Galt heard a rumor that some members of the staff had given up two weeks of their rations to feed the hungry patients. On April 16 Wager, who later said he bought supplies for a few days on credit in the neighborhood, wrote to the medical director of the Fourth United

States Army Corps at Yorktown that unless speedy relief was sent "the patients *must Starve*." General Wise wanted Wager to run the hospital and would aid in every way possible. Three officers had left, and "four of the Servants have been taken away, & nearly all the rest have absconded." He, Wager, was treated with every consideration, but "in the name of humanity" the army must send at least ten days' provisions.

The Union command, angry at the treatment as prisoners of war of the two cavalrymen "acting as nurses to the insane—to those whom Governor Wise styled Virginia's 'little ones' and as belonging to a 'hospital the most exempt of all from the least touch of war,' " ordered Wager on the sixteenth to withdraw from the Confederate lines, that is, to leave the hospital. He did so the next day. There was thus a sort of interregnum at the hospital. For the some 250 patients "there was *no control* at all, not even to restrain [them] within the limits of the asylum." It was "in a great degree destitute of officers, servants, provisions, and other usual and necessary appendages."

Wise thought the order to withdraw Wager, which was sent to his headquarters, a trick, probably to discover his intentions. He ordered a staff officer not to acknowledge it, as he "had anticipated some such ruse, and yesterday had arranged with Talbot Sweeny [*sic*] esq., the only State of Virginia officer left with the asylum, to attend to and provide for its wants." Wise also would send Dr. William Martin, a local physician, "to superintend its hygeia." On April 17 Wise gave the keys of the asylum to Sweeney, who considered himself temporarily in charge since the directors "for reasons satisfactory to the Government of Virginia [were] absent from their post of duty." Sweeney then appointed a staff, including several former employees.

Wise's concern that he not be blamed for the hospital's plight is shown in his letter to Dr. Martin who, afraid, had refused to come there. Martin would be safe, Wise wrote, as the Federal and Confederate governments had an arrangement that physicians and surgeons working in hospitals were not to be treated as prisoners of war. Wise, "anxious that the enemy shall not have it to say that we abandoned the cure and care of our own patients," begged

Martin to take charge of the hospital: "Force them to turn you out."

Meanwhile the patients were starving and Wise could not provision them. So on the 17th he sent Sweeney, Major John D. Munford (a hospital director) and two others to the Union lines to ask Colonel Robert M. West, commander of Fort Magruder, for help. He also asked for Federal protection of the personnel and property "of those Institutions required to provide for and nurse the sick and the infirm." The hospital staff would be under "Parole of Honor" to "communicate nothing to damage the Fedl Forces," but not to be considered prisoners of war. By then Wise had withdrawn above Williamsburg and the hospital was under no one's control. General E. D. Keyes, West's superior and commander of the Fourth Army Corps at Yorktown, when told the patients were "on the borders of absolute starvation," ordered ten days' rations for them and sent back the paroled attendants.

Sweeney wrote Wise that he had accepted an offer of supplies from West. Wise should hold on if he could for a few more days, Sweeney advised, and "make what demonstration [he thought] best before the Town," but should guard his flanks, as it was difficult to tell what the Federals were after. West's conduct during the interview, however, was, in justice to him, exemplary. At the same time, Sweeney wondered if his committee would be compromised by taking the supplies. Indeed not, Wise replied. Certainly Wise himself could not enter into such an agreement, and the patients should not be allowed to suffer. Sweeney might properly not only accept but as legal adviser of the asylum claim the supplies already there or intended for it.

West, however, in acceding to Wise's terms, including a guarantee of protection for the hospital and its personnel, had exceeded his authority. His commander would not sustain him, so Sweeney must write to the latter for such assurances. But, Sweeney wrote, West would supply the hospital with the supplies at Fort Magruder intended for it, "from a sincere motive to help the afflicted patients (and which *assurance we believed then, as we do now*)." Sweeney and his committee accepted the provisions "in the same humane spirit." At this point West declared that "in this matter he would not be outdone by any person in generosity."

The Union position was more or less officially communicated to the Confederates in a letter from General Keyes's assistant adjutant general to the chief quartermaster of his corps, a copy of which was given to Sweeney so that Wise might "learn in what estimation he was held." Keyes, the letter said, was "informed that notwithstanding the late occupation of Williamsburg by the rebel forces under General Wise and the consequent abandonment of the city by the Union troops," no provision was made for the support of the inmates of the asylum, tenanted as it was "by their own kith and kin and by a class of patients demanding of all the civilized world the tenderest care and solicitude."

Keyes was "not willing that the imputation of inhumanity and want of civilization, so justly chargeable to these traitors to their counry and enemies of their own blood, should rest, even with the lightest touch of seeming truth, upon himself or those in his command as representing in this section of the country the dignity and care of the Government of the United States." Therefore, despite the reprehensible actions of the Confederates and the fact that the town of Williamsburg and the asylum were not occupied by the Union forces and were beyond their picket lines, "in the name of humanity and Christianity," the commanding general directed that a ten-days' supply of rations for 250 men be sent at once to the asylum for the inmates.

Wise defended himself in an emotional letter, containing some inaccuracies, to Sweeney and his committee. He had advanced on the Federals at Williamsburg on April 11, under "purely military orders," planning to pass through and attack Fort Magruder. He had intended not to take charge of or provide for any civil institutions, only to defend them from "the ruthless invaders" who "had seized and occupied the Town of Williamsburg . . . burnt her most ancient College . . . driven from her Asylum for the insane its superintendent, its surgeons, its matron and nurses, and by force of arms had cut off all approaches of supplies to its wants, and had assumed all the responsibilities due to humanity in behalf of the sick and insane." They placed their own staff in charge and undertook to provide for the inmates of the hospital.

In any case, Wise wrote, the country was so ravaged that its citizens could not supply the needs of such a large institution, especially when the Federals had restricted their movements. As for the Confederate forces, their first obligation was to drive the "invader" back, not to worry about the sick or insane. "They had to *fight,* not to *nurse.*" What if the asylum was abandoned? It was only an encumbrance, and what guarantee was there that if it was again supplied it would not again be disturbed, its personnel turned out, and its provisions seized?

Under these circumstances Wise had declined to interfere with the asylum at all; he had no orders to do so. He had left the town to save it from shelling, "to preserve the Asylum and its quiet, and to give the invader the fair opportunity of testing with superior force who should & who should not be the guardians of our own people, both the healthy and infirm." Therefore he had assured Wager and all the asylum personnel of protection on condition that they not divulge any Confederate intelligence to the Union forces. "But it was found that several of the servants & nurses were fugitive slaves, belonging to masters who claimed their private property, and they were allowed to take them away."

The letter sent by Keyes's adjutant was "as false in fact as it is affected in sentiment," its motives obviously those of "military spleen & political chicanery, not of humanity or common charity." Wise told Sweeney to repel any protection offered; he had "already *inquired* in vain" whether the Federals would "seize the asylum or allow it again to be molested." Despite the risks, Sweeney should take charge of the hospital and for the patients' sake accept all the provisions that the Federals would furnish, "without any guarantees of protection, and notwithstanding their air of arrogance and patronage." Wise also advised that the whole matter be reported immediately to the governor so that he might "make some satisfactory arrangements."

Wise himself wrote to Governor Letcher in Richmond asking the state authorities to make "without delay, the necessary arrangements for providing rations, fuel &c" for the asylum, as the military could give no aid. Sweeney also asked the governor for advice. Since the old officers had abandoned the institution he would have to appoint temporary replacements, but would do nothing to embarrass the governor in case the Federal forces reoccupied the town. Sweeney would be "governed solely by a sincere interest in the welfare of the inmates, and the honour of Va." Did the governor authorize entering into any understanding with the Union command which would secure to him the control of the asylum whether or not the Union troops reoccupied Williamsburg? Or would the governor think it best to throw upon the Federals the responsibility of the institution along with their occupation of the town?

The fast moving events caught Letcher in an embarrassing position. He could not directly help the hospital and in any case had no authority to do so, and he feared that the Union forces would not afford it the "protection desired." Therefore, on the advice of Saunders he was sending to Williamsburg the former steward, Douglas, to take charge of the hospital. The latter, as the legal representative of the board, could legitimately provide for the inmates and draw on state money. Letcher hoped Wise would do all he could to secure protection of the institution and put Douglas in touch with the Federal authorities.

In a brief description of the whole business to his commanding officer, Wise gave a version somewhat different from that in his letter to Sweeney and the others:

> The Yankee rascals tried to throw the hospital on my hands to embarrass and pump me as to my purpose of permanent occupation. I declined to have anything to do with it, and they retired their superintendent, nurses, &c. I then gave it up to the State civil authorities who by my counsel, obtained for them ten days' provisions, without compromising our dignity or claiming from them any protection. . . . You may assure the Governor that the patients will not suffer as I know they will take charge of the Asylum again now that I have retired.

Williamsburg and Fort Magruder, though not in the hands of the Confederates, were still subject to their attack and therefore not secure for the Union forces. But the continued harassment by Wise's guerrillas actually hurt the residents of Williamsburg and especially the patients at the hospital more than it damaged the Union army. General John A. Dix, Keyes's superior and commanding officer of the Department of Virginia at Fort Monroe, understood these difficulties and made the most of them.

In a long letter he complained to Wise about the raids on Williamsburg, actions designed not to hold the town or take over the hospital but only to harass the Federals and for no good military purpose. Many of the inhabitants were known not to be well disposed to the United States government, yet they had been unmolested and allowed to pursue their "domestic avocations" and procure goods at Yorktown and Fort Monroe. The asylum had been provisioned and put under the superintendence of an army surgeon. The actions of Wise's men when they entered the town deprived the hospital's inmates of the care to which they were accustomed and which their helpless condition rendered indispensable. By withdrawing his forces Wise again left the hospital "to our charity" and compelled Keyes to supply it with food "to save the patients from starvation."

These raids, therefore, violated "every dictate of humanity" and "every principle of honorable warfare." Dix had directed Keyes to reoccupy the town and threatened that if the raids recurred the hospital inmates would be sent to Richmond, any house used for firing at Federal troops would be razed to the ground, and any citizen of Williamsburg not belonging to a regular organized corps who was found cooperating in the raids and rising in arms against the Federals would be executed as "a violator of the laws of civilized warfare."

The Union commanders, though better able to supply the hospital than were either Wise's troops or the townspeople, also felt it an encumbrance and were not sure what to do with it. "Do you think it would be advisable for us to let the Confederates take charge of the insane asylum?" Dix asked Keyes a few days after he had written to Wise. "They would be sending in and going out for supplies and it seems to me it would be a means of communication with the rebels. Douglass [*sic*] can come back as steward, if you think proper, under our superintendence." Keyes thought the case of the asylum difficult no matter who controlled it. If in Confederate hands, "it would afford a standing pretext for visits from their emissaries, which evil must be balanced by our troubles with the institution. I would like to have you decide the question. Douglass [*sic*] I regard as a pretty bad rebel."

Dix did not yield the hospital either to the Confederates or to Douglas, but his letter to Wise must have struck home. Williamsburg was no longer troubled by raiders or snipers, so that life could return to something like normal, under control of Union pickets and a provost marshal. The hospital remained under unofficial command of the Union army and provisioned by it, with Sweeney in charge and his staff serving without pay until February 1864. At that time Wager was again ordered to act as superintendent, the hospital thus being placed directly under the official supervision of the United States Army until the fall of 1865.

Practically everyone who discussed the fate of the hospital during the crises of 1862 and 1863 did so in terms of the cure as well as the care of the patients and in the context of humanitarianism and Christianity, each side vying for the honors of civilized behavior. The military commanders—Wise, Dix, Keyes, West (two of whom, Dix and Wise, were well-known statesmen and politicians in civilian life)—spoke of the hospital as a therapeutic institution and maintained that they acted out of the highest motives of humanity and honor. This contest, even if not as moralistic as presented, did result in the hospital's being provisioned and in inducing both sides to treat the insane better perhaps than might have been expected. And always, though most of the staff and board members left at the first sign of danger, a few persons remained, sometimes only one, to worry enough about the patients that at least they were fed.

[4]

By all reports, Wager conducted the asylum fairly well, especially since he probably had never treated mental patients before. The extant records of the hospital contain various orders of admissions, discharges, registers of patients, case records, and other information indicating that Wager was conscientious in his duties. The number of admissions was small, only five in 1862 and again in 1863, rising to thirteen in 1864 and thirty-six in 1865. Low admissions, many deaths, some recoveries, and a few escapes caused the patient population to drop, so that when Wager returned in February 1864 there were only 183 and by October 31, 1865, when he surrendered the hospital to civilian authorities, 180 patients, compared to some 250 in 1863.

Wager may have discharged some patients before they were wholly restored. If so, this was was probably more from inexperience than incompetence; the records show that each discharge followed an examination of the patient by Wager as to his sanity. The patients came from both occupied and unoccupied sections of Virginia and included blacks and whites, soldiers and civilians. Discharged patients occasionally had to find their own way home without funds or provisions, but it seems that attempts were made to have them sent home safely even if they lived within the Confederate lines.

Wager's primary efforts at the hospital, one suspects, were to take care of the patients' physical and essential medical needs. His staff numbered fifty-five ward officers and attendants, including several experienced former officers, who were paid by the United States Army from 1864 until the end of October 1865. Shortly after Wager returned as superintendent he requisitioned a long list of medicines, hospital stores, dressings, and other medical supplies from the army, thus indicating both the needs at the hospital and his own medical orientation.

How much the various practices of moral treatment were continued under his administration is unknown, but surely very little. Through all the vicissitudes of the war the most important aim was physical survival, though during the Sweeney interregnum in 1863 Sally Galt wrote that the patients were "generally well" and came to see her every two or three days. They borrowed books and she gave them flowers from her garden. Soon after Wager returned she went to hear preaching in the ladies' parlor. The patients "seemed to like it exceedingly & all looked very bright and happy."

Wager had a good reputation in Williamsburg, notwithstanding his being a northern soldier and an alcoholic. After his death in

1868 (of acute alcoholism) the assistant physician and acting superintendent of the asylum wrote of his "many noble characteristics and generous impulses [which] won for him the esteem & affection of many of the best citizens," who knew his foibles but were willing "to throw the vail [*sic*] of charity over his memory."

Sally Galt evidently developed good relations with him, much as it may have pained her to see a stranger, and a Union army officer at that, filling John Minson Galt II's place. She even gave him a book on surgery from her brother's library, an act inconceivable on her part if Wager had treated the patients badly or herself with less than due respect. Wager thanked her graciously: he would "ever fondly cherish [the book] in remembrance of the Source from whence it came, & as having been the property of a most estimable & exemplary gentleman."

The role of Dorothea Dix in the hospital's affairs during the war is not altogether clear. Sally Galt erred in saying that she was placed in charge of the hospital by President Lincoln in June 1862. However, Miss Dix, whose duties as superintendent of women nurses for the Union forces took her frequently to Washington and Fort Monroe, did show a special interest in the asylum and in Miss Galt, still grief-stricken and upset by her brother's death and the events of the war. In 1863 Miss Dix visited the hospital, to the delight of the patients, to whom she sent presents of tobacco, paper, and laces. It also gave them joy to see Sally Galt, whom Miss Dix had persuaded to resume contact with the asylum in order to do what she could for the patients.

Early in 1864 Miss Galt, afraid she would have to take an oath of loyalty to the United States government, frantically begged Miss Dix for help. Otherwise she might be turned out of her house and out of Williamsburg. In her emotional letters to Miss Dix and to the local commanding officers she declared that she would take an oath to no government; one officer interpreted her refusal as nonpolitical, rather that of a "religious recluse." (From various other letters written to friends during the war, it is clear that she was a staunch Confederate.) Miss Dix probably did intercede; whether through her doing or Miss Galt's appeals, or both, the military commanders excused Miss Galt from taking the oath and ordered that she be allowed to remain where she was, without molestation.

Miss Galt also asked Miss Dix's help in being allowed to give to the asylum her house and garden, in case she should have to leave, including John Minson Galt II's library, his collection of rare shells and curiosities, and a marble bust of him. Miss Dix approved and apparently interceded with General Butler to obtain his consent. Miss Galt was so grateful, she wrote:

> The thought will be comforting to me, that the flowers will bloom & the fruit will ripen in the dear 'Old Garden' for the Patients. . . . Perhaps it is better for the patients to enjoy it, than to own it myself, for it may be a restorative measure to walk in this sweet garden. I think all writers on Insanity agree as to the useful influences of change of scene & exercise in pleasure grounds. I know this was the opinion of my Darling Brother.

She was recently at the hospital and "you can't think how ornamental my pictures are; some of them are hung in the sleeping rooms, of those who can appreciate a picture. I ought to love the Asylum, for not very long after its commencement 84 years ago, my grandfather Dr. John M. Galt was appointed Surgeon."

Her house and garden did not go to the hospital (though she may have sent the library there temporarily for safekeeping) probably because despite all the desperate fighting then near Richmond and Petersburg Miss Galt could remain at home safely. Her will made in 1869 bequeathed only her brother's psychiatric library, museum, and marble bust to the hospital; it received after her death in 1880 only the bust (Figure 10).

Miss Dix came to the aid of the asylum in September 1865 in response to urgent pleas from Miss Galt that the patients were greatly in need of supplies. By this time the war was over, and the re-establishment of civilian authority in Virginia under the Union administration of Governor Pierpont created a problem of proper requisitioning. In June the General Assembly authorized the governor to draw money from the treasury as needed to defray the expenses of the Eastern and Western State hospitals and the Institu-

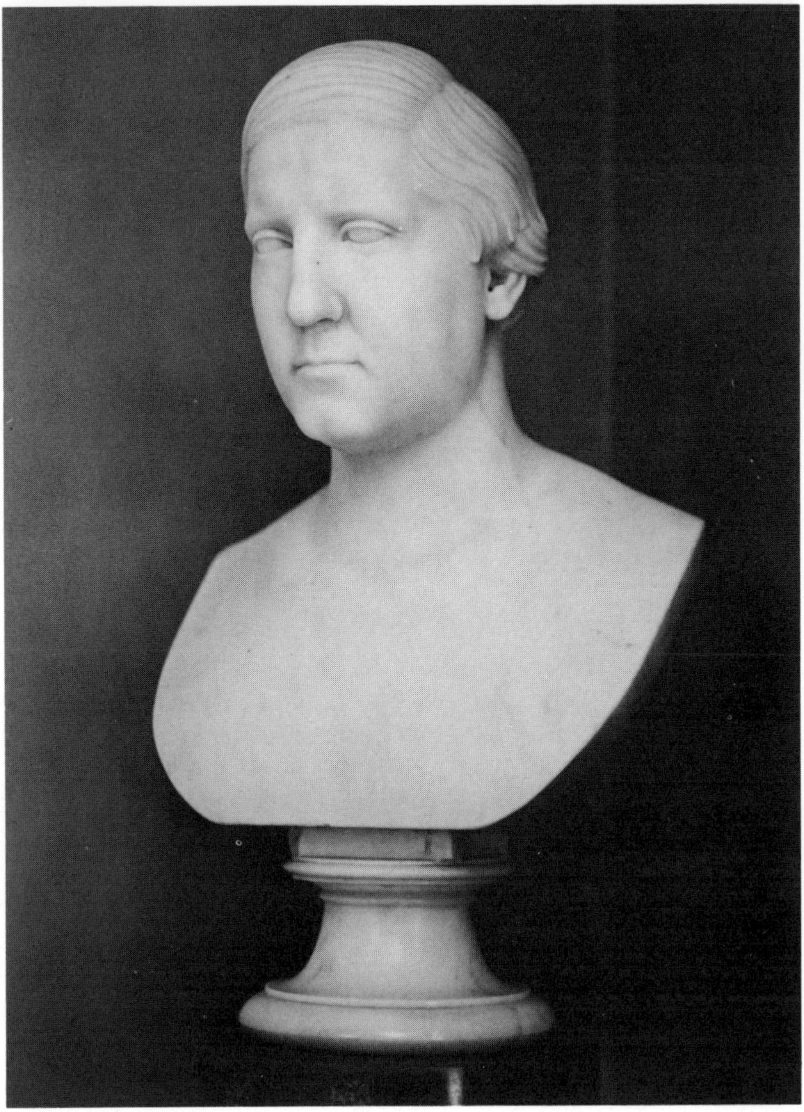

Figure 11
Bust of John Minson Galt II

The sculptor was probably a Norfolk cousin, Alexander Galt (1827–1863), whose best known work is the marble statue of Thomas Jefferson at the University of Virginia. (Photograph by Thomas L. Williams, courtesy of Eastern State Hospital.)

tion for the Deaf-Dumb and Blind for the current year. At the same time the United States Army authorities were anxious to have the state assume charge of the hospital, "thus relieving the Government [of the United States] of an expense of at least fifty thousand ($50,000) a year." On September 12 Pierpont appointed a board of directors for the hospital as of November 1. Included on the board were Lemuel G. Bowden, son of Lemuel J. Bowden who died in 1864, and only one other man from Williamsburg. This would make it difficult for the board to meet regularly to transact the hospital's business and decide on admissions and discharges of patients.

The new board wanted to take over the hospital immediately, but Wager, though willing to give it up, could not do so without orders from his superiors. On October 14 the board authorized its newly elected president, Lemuel G. Bowden, and another director, Dr. C. M. Hubbard (elected assistant physician as of his resignation from the board), to see the governor and the military authorities at Richmond to "urge the necessity of turning the Asylum over to the State authorities, in view of the present deplorable condition of the unfortunate insane at this place."

Bowden wrote to Pierpont asking that Wager be removed "for the sake of the dignity of the State and for the sake of humanity." Wager's refusal to turn over the hospital was insulting to the board and to the state whose authority he did not recognize. Further, Wager had "on three or four occasions during the present year been confined to his room or bed by the *Mania aportu* (drunkenness) one of which attacks lasted for over a month, during which time the unforunate insane were left in the hands of inexperienced nurses and without any medical attendance"; since the war ended several patients had been removed from the asylum by relatives, "simply from the reason of their treatment."

Perhaps so. Wager did drink to excess, but nowhere else was it said that he neglected patients. He testified in 1866 that the new board, on inspecting the hospital in October 1865, "expressed themselves highly gratified at its condition," Dr. Hubbard, a frequent visitor, stating "that he had never known it in a better condition than under the administration of [Wager]." Because of the ambiguity and uncertainty about jurisdiction over the hospital, however, Wager did delay requesting needed provisions, so that the patients were suffering, especially from lack of clothing and medical stores. By November 1 there was food enough for only one meal; the patients were "dressed in all they had and the clothes room [was] entirely depleted."

Finally on October 31 Wager, having received orders to do so, surrendered the hospital to the board. In his letter of transfer he said he had requisitioned from the quartermaster general the necessary supplies for the coming winter. Miss Dix, seriously uneasy about the patients with the cold season coming on, had written to him and had also communicated with the secretary of war, who ordered the quartermaster general of the army to supply the hospital. The board did not accept these goods, since they were received after Wager left and when therefore the hospital was again in civilian hands; further, the "urgent necessities" of the patients demanded more "immediate action." Instead they obtained an emergency appropriation of $15,000 from the state.

[5]

One of the first acts of the board, aside from trying to establish its jurisdiction over the hospital and appointing several of its own members to lucrative positions, was to pass a resolution eulogizing John Minson Galt II, copies of which were to be sent to the Williamsburg and Richmond papers. The board also proceeded to appoint a staff, many of them old officers, and put the asylum on a going basis. The hospital needed not only food, clothing, and medicines for the patients but also rehabilitation. The first postwar annual report described it as being in a "debilitated and deranged condition," with bad drainage of waste and sewage, poor lighting, gasworks and laundry machinery out of order, and inadequate heating facilities. The main buildings, however, had survived the war well and needed few repairs.

But attention was soon directed to the conduct of the board. The old struggles over spoils and patronage that had plagued the Eastern State Hospital before the war quickly reappeared, with the added feature of pro- and anti-Unionist factions fighting for control and trying to discredit each other. The affairs of the hospital went into an "interminable broil." The board consisted of many Unionists, including its president Lemuel G. Bowden, brother of the attorney general of the state and nephew of Henry Bowden, then living in Norfolk and presumably an active Republican.

The first charges against the directors came from a staff member at the hospital who said he had lost his job, as others had, because he did not vote for Lemuel G. Bowden as a delegate to the state legislature. Charges that the hospital was used for political patronage reached the General Assembly and the governor. In December 1865 the assembly heard a resolution to investigate the conduct of the Williamsburg hospital during the war and its current management; there were also proposals to investigate the Staunton hospital.

After various maneuverings the General Assembly decided to look into the affairs of the two asylums; on January 16, 1866, an investigating committee heard testimony in Williamsburg. Only a few days before, Governor Pierpont had sent a letter to the Senate and House informing the members that he had heard of "certain irregularities in the conduct of the board of directors of the lunatic asylum at Williamsburg." He asked the legislature to investigate "all matters connected with the institutions wherein the state has had representatives since the 1st of June 1850." He, as governor, had not the requisite power to do anything about the matter.

Various former and present directors and officers of the Eastern State Hospital, including Henry Bowden and Dr. Wager, gave depositions to the investigating committee. The two major issues concerned the wartime management of the hospital, especially the behavior of Dr. Watson and Henry Bowden when they left in August 1862 with the hospital's supplies, and the alleged use of the hospital's patronage for political purposes by the postwar board. Saunders and Sweeney also made statements supporting the claims of staff members for salaries due them for work during the war. Testimony naturally varied, partly with the political sympathies of the deponents. The proceedings are valuable, nevertheless, in connection with extant records of the war years themselves, in piecing together the events of 1862–1865.

The investigating committee reported that the asylum's supplies and money were "improperly used or disposed of without being accounted for" during the war and that its records were mutilated and minutes taken away by Henry Bowden, who still had them. The directors of the hospital should hold responsible the persons who did this and seek restitution, by law if necessary. As for the current management, some of the board had used the patronage and offices of the asylum "for party and political purposes." Lemuel G. Bowden held the federal office of assistant tax collector, which not only took him away from Williamsburg but vacated his office of director. Several of the directors lived too far away to participate in the business of the hospital, so that a quorum was difficult to gather. Consequently the superintendent was illegally passing on the admission and discharge of patients and attending to the asylum's business, much of which was left undone.

The committee demanded "a radical change in the administration of the asylum." Otherwise its usefulness would be destroyed, and instead of "being a home and a hospital for the cure and maintenance of our unfortunate fellow-creatures," it would continue to be made a machine to be used, by those having its control, to reward friends or purchase office. This reform would be effected by a change of directors, which the committee recommended to the governor, who appointed a new board. Claims against the state for supplies and salaries during the war were recognized in a law appropriating $18,336.55 to provide for the hospital's liabilities incurred before July 1, 1865.

The new board named by the governor in February 1866 contained mainly local men, including several prewar directors and officers, among them W. W. Vest, who became president. Dr. Leonard Henley, the superintendent, refused to recognize this body and would not admit them to the hospital grounds. Undaunted, they met in the local Baptist church and, following precedent faithfully, proceeded to elect some of their number to profitable positions. One, the former assistant and then consulting physician, Robert M. Garrett, was named superintendent and resigned as director, finally achieving the post he had wanted during Galt's time. Word of these actions reached the legislature, which initiated another investigation in order to complete the first one and because the new board was proving as bad as the old.

Thus began a new round of investigations, charges, defenses, and countercharges. Superintendents and members of the board came and went in rapid succession, usually if not always under a justified accusation of malfeasance in office. For an interim period in 1868/69, government by the United States Army superseded a board dissolved on account of corruption. The patients for the most part fared indifferently. Occasionally a superintendent during these years made serious efforts to reconstitute the Eastern State Hospital as a therapeutic institution, with temporary success. By the 1870s conditions were still unstable. The impoverished Sally Galt, asking Dorothea Dix for help in getting a job at a mental hospital, wrote,

> You will naturally enquire . . . why I don't get a position in our Asylum. There are no Female offices vacant & perhaps I may not like to serve where I have resided. Also nothing is stable here, 13 or 14 medical superintendents have been installed since 1862 & 6 of them since the war broke up. Just now we have a most efficient & excellent superintendent from Penn. Dr. Brower. But in the dear Old Dominion all is in a state of abeyance nothing permanent, nothing settled.

Sally Galt did not leave Williamsburg to work in a mental hospital, nor did affairs at the Eastern State Hospital settle down in her lifetime. As in its earlier history that institution continued to suffer the fate of the society it served, a sociey that would for years feel the disruptions of the war. The administration of John Minson Galt II, however flawed, long remained for the Eastern State Hospital a pinnacle of accomplishment.

A Note on the Sources

WHEN this study was first proposed there was a question whether the extant sources would be adequate for more than a superficial history of the Eastern State Hospital. Many records were thought to have been destroyed during the Civil War, and as the hospital was fairly obscure there was not extensive mention of it in published works. Aside from a few sketchy articles on the history of the hospital, the most substantial work on the subject consisted of two unpublished master's theses completed at the College of William and Mary: "A History of the Eastern State Hospital of Virginia under the Galt Family (1773–1862)," by James Harding Siske (1949) and "A Brief History of the Eastern State Hospital as Shown by a Study of the Early Records of the Hospital," by Esther Garland Iglehart (1930). Unfortunately these essays, based as they were on limited research, did not deal with many important issues.

Fuller investigation of the sources yielded a great deal of significant material—much more than had been assumed to exist. Consequently I saw that, with certain gaps, a serious study of the hospital and those who served it could be undertaken. Much historical research is something of a detective story, and the leads followed often reveal more surprises than the average whodunit. In this case a wide variety of sources could be utilized to piece together what turned out to be in some respects a unique story, one that adds a new dimension to our understanding of the history of mental illness and its treatment in the United States, particularly in the South. A copy of the fully documented manuscript of this book is on deposit at Colonial Williamsburg and available for reference.

The richest and most absorbing source is the collection of Galt Family Papers on deposit with Colonial Williamsburg and used by permission of the Galt descendants. These papers include over five thousand items, most of which relate to the physicians who worked at the hospital. They contain personal and medical papers, memorabilia, and a file of the published writings of Dr. John Minson Galt II. Many hundreds of letters to and from the Galt physicians and their families, friends, and professional colleagues furnish a composite picture of the Galts, their relations with the hospital, life at the hospital, and the social and political atmosphere of Williamsburg. There are also the personal and medical diaries of Dr. Alexander D. Galt and his son, Dr. John Minson Galt II; these are very frank and obviously not written for publication as were so many diaries composed in the nineteenth century. J. M. Galt II's personal diary is quite extensive, spanning almost his entire adult life (from 1838 to 1859) and revealing his personality and intellectual development as well as his emotional problems. His medical diary (1851–1855)) tells us less about medical matters than about administrative and political affairs at the hospital. For the earlier years the hospital notes kept by Drs. John Minson Galt I and Philip Barraud (1799–1809) describe medical practices, and A. D. Galt's medical diary does the same for the 1830s; J. M. Galt II's case histories (1841–1845) provide some specific examples of patient care during the first years of his administration. Valuable but not always accurate are the biographical sketches in Sally Galt's hand (some of them written by other persons) of her father, grandfather, and brother. These writings express family traditions about the hospital from Revolutionary times.

Other vital records are the minutes of the Court of Directors of the hospital. They were kept irregularly and are incomplete. Those for the period from December 10, 1770 to July 23, 1801 are in the Virginia State Library and available in photostatic copies at Colonial Williamsburg; the present Eastern State Hospital has in its archives the minutes from 1822 to 1866 (and beyond). Those for mid-1801 through 1821 are missing. During the Civil War the board did not meet for several years though Union officers kept sporadic notes in the minute book. The minutes contain a broad range of information on all aspects of the hospital's administration and operation (including data on each patient committed and discharged) and are an official record of the directors' activities and decisions. In the hospital's archives are also a few other manuscripts such as lists of patients, case histories for scattered years, and several letters and drafts of reports by John Minson Galt II.

In 1822 the General Assembly of Virginia required the directors of the Eastern State Hospital to submit annual reports on the condition of the hospital. They were usually printed in the *Journal* of the House of Delegates and in 1841 were ordered to be published separately as well. Hence these are a convenient source of statistics and other data about the hospital year by year. In addition to information on various aspects of the hospital's administration, J. M. Galt II chose to include in the reports his theories about mental illness and its proper treatment, hoping thereby to educate legislators and the general public. The reports aid greatly in understanding some of the problems the hospital faced and Galt's solutions of them.

A large body of laws and other public documents relating to the hospital are in the Virginia State Library, the Law library of the College of William and Mary, and the Research Department of Colonial Williamsburg. Some of these documents are of great importance, for example, laws founding the hospital and regulating its affairs, reports of legislative investigating committees, and governors' speeches. The pre-Revolutionary journals of the House of Burgesses and the Council of Virginia and those of the subsequent House of Delegates and Senate record legislative action and debate concerning the hospital. The *Calendar of Virginia State Papers* include a number of relevant documents and letters, as do other published collections of official papers. The State Archives in the State Library contain a variety of records pertaining to the hospital, the most valuable being those in the Executive Papers and collections of petitions to the Assembly.

Much of the material mentioned thus far is richer for the nineteenth than for the eighteenth century. A large and scattered group of sources had to be searched in order to reconstruct events during the early period; the same was true for the Civil War years. Most helpful for the colonial, Revolutionary, and post-Revolutionary years were the extensive resources of Colonial Williamsburg's

Research Department where materials of all kinds pertaining to eighteenth-century Williamsburg and Virginia have been brought together. Besides books, articles, and microfilms of manuscripts there are data files, research query files, and typescript copies of memoirs of Williamsburg residents. Among these is a detailed account of the town during the Civil War, "The Vest Mansion, Its Historical and Romantic Associations as Confederate and Union Headquarters (1862–1865) in the American Civil War," by David Edward Cronin, a Union officer and provost marshal of Williamsburg in 1864. Several reports prepared by Research Department staff members hold interesting information. For example, Harold B. Gill, Jr.'s "The Apothecary in Colonial America" (1963) supplies data on local pharmacological practices as well as biographical material on John Minson Galt I. Gill's "The Blacksmith in Colonial Virginia" (1965) includes in the records of a local blacksmith the fact that chains and leg irons were made for the hospital late in the eighteenth century. Another report, "The Eastern State Hospital at Williamsburg, Virginia" (1950) brings together most of the extant illustrations of the hospital, including copies of insurance policies that for the nineteenth century show the position of the buildings on the grounds. A section in Marcus Whiffen's *The Public Buildings of Williamsburg* (Williamsburg, 1958) is devoted to the hospital and includes a reconstruction of the plan of the first building.

At the College of William and Mary, the Eastern State Hospital Collection contains miscellaneous papers, and the Southall Papers are revealing about the political and economic struggles for control at the hospital during the early 1850s. The Virginia Historical Society has a genealogical chart of the Galt family, which, while not entirely accurate, is extremely useful (together with family histories published by several Galts and others). There is also in the society a memoir relating to the hospital during the Civil War. The Military Records Division of the National Archives yielded valuable information about the hospital in the war years, especially for the period during which Dr. Peter Wager, the Union officer, was in charge.

Several important items appeared in the Lincoln Papers at the Library of Congress, and the United States War Department's *War of the Rebellion* includes correspondence pertaining to the hospital during 1862 and 1863.

Quite unexpected was the discovery of a large collection of letters at the Western State Hospital at Staunton that have significance beyond this study. Among them is correspondence not only beween Francis Stribling and John M. Galt II but also between Stribling and Dorothea L. Dix and many well-known psychiatrists of their day. These letters were fortunately saved from the fire to which old hospital records had been consigned after being microfimed. The extensive microfilmed records include correspondence between Stribling and Galt and between Stribling and state legislators relating to the Eastern and Western State hospitals' dispute over territorial jurisdiction. These documents supplement the memoranda and letters on that controversy to be found in the Galt Family Papers and in the board minutes of the Eastern State Hospital. The microfilms also reveal a multitude of letters to Stribling from patients and friends, providing—as do Western State's published annual reports—further basis for comparing the two institutions.

Newspapers were used selectively, especially for the nineteenth century. The *Virginia Gazette Index, 1736–1780* (eds. Lester J. Cappon and Stella F. Duff, 1950) provided a number of useful references. For subsequent years adequate newspaper indexes do not exist, so that a thorough search for items about the hospital or about mental illness, even in one newspaper, was not practicable. The newspaper collection at the Virginia State Library could only be investigated for specific dates or short periods of time when the papers might be expected to discuss hospital affairs. The *Richmond Enquirer* yielded editorial comments, news items, and proceedings of legislative debates particularly helpful in analyzing hospital affairs during the early 1850s. E. G. Swem's *Virginia Historical Index* (1934) is invaluable in searching nineteenth-century and later periodical publications as well as the *Calendar of Virginia State Papers* and Hening's *Statutes of Virginia*. Of the historical magazines indexed in Swem the most important for this study were the *William and Mary Quarterly*, *Tyler's Quarterly Historical and Genealogical Magazine* and the *Virginia Magazine of History and Biography*, all of which published many pertinent primary records.

I have mentioned for the most part only the major primary sources consulted. A number of other manuscript collections, such as the Kirkbride Papers at the Pennsylvania Hospital, various papers at the University of Virginia, and the Dorothea Dix Papers at Harvard University, also furnished material, as did early periodicals at the Medical College of Virginia. I also drew on my own previous extensive research in the psychiatric and medical literature of the mid-eighteenth through the mid-nineteenth centuries.

The several historical articles written about the hospital are brief and scarcely make an original contribution to the subject. Indeed, there has been published in the secondary historical literature relatively little that is worthwhile on American mental hospitals and mental illness, and the few books and articles of merit mainly, though not exclusively, treat northern institutions and conditions. A standard older work is Henry M. Hurd, ed., *The Institutional Care of the Insane in the United States and Canada*, 4 vols. (Baltimore, 1916). Some of the more recent studies that reflect a new interest in the history of mental illness are Albert Deutsch's classic *The Mentally Ill in America: A History of Their Care and Treatment from Colonial Times*, 2d ed., rev. and enl. (New York, 1949); the American Psychiatric Association's collection of articles, *One Hundred Years of American Psychiatry* (New York, 1944); *New England Hospitals, 1790–1833*, by Leonard K. Eaton (Ann Arbor, 1957); and Norman Dain, *Concepts of Insanity in the United States, 1789–1865* (New Brunswick, N. J., 1964). Several specialized works offer bases for comparison with the Eastern State Hospital: William Logie Russell, *The New York Hospital: A History of the Psychiatric Service, 1771–1936* (New York, 1945); Gerald N. Grob, *The State and the Mentally Ill: A History of Worcester State Hospital in Massachusetts, 1830–1920* (Chapel Hill, 1966); and James Leiby, *Charity and Correction in New Jersey; A History of State Welfare Institutions* (New Brunswick, N. J., 1967). There are also various articles in the *Bulletin of the History of Medicine*, the *American Journal of Psychiatry*, the *Journal of Nervous and Mental Disease*, and elsewhere that are cited in the documented original manuscript of this book.

Index

———
*Eastern State Hospital